D1111756

TAKING
CONTROL
of
TMJ

Your Total Wellness
Program for Recovering from
Temporomandibular Joint Pain,
Whiplash, Fibromyalgia,
and Related Disorders

ROBERT O. UPPGAARD, D.D.S.

New Harbinger Publications

Publisher's Note

This publication is designed to provide accurate and authoritative information in regard to the subject matter covered. It is sold with the understanding that the publisher is not engaged in rendering psychological, financial, legal, or other professional services. If expert assistance or counseling is needed, the services of a competent professional should be sought.

Distributed in the U.S.A. by Publishers Group West; in Canada by Raincoast Books; in Great Britain by Airlift Book Company, Ltd.; in South Africa by Real Books, Ltd.; in Australia by Boobook; and in New Zealand by Tandem Press.

Copyright © 1999 by Robert O. Uppgaard, D.D.S.
New Harbinger Publications, Inc.
5674 Shattuck Avenue
Oakland, CA 94609

Cover design © 1998 by Lightbourne Images
Text design by Michele Waters

Library of Congress Catalog Card Number: 98-67409
ISBN 1-57224-126-8 Paperback

All Rights Reserved

Printed in the United States of America on recycled paper

New Harbinger Publications' Website address: www.newharbinger.com

01   00   99

10   9   8   7   6   5   4   3   2

Not until diagnosis becomes the foundation on which the whole structure of dentistry is built can it lay claim to be a learned profession or an important branch of the great art and science of healing.

Leroy M. S. Miner, D.D.S.

Contents

Foreword   *vii*

Acknowledgments   *ix*

Introduction   *1*

Part I
Your Total Wellness Program

1   Understand the Problem   *11*

2   Exercises to Improve Jaw Functioning   *35*

3   Treat Referred Pain from Trigger Points   *45*

4   Eliminate Harmful Habits   *59*

5   Identify Stressors   *81*

6   Evaluate and Improve Diet and Exercise Habits   *95*

Part II
Other Considerations in Taking Control of TMJ

7   Whiplash and TMJ Disorder   *121*

8   Fibromyalgia and TMJ Disorder   *133*

9   Splints   *141*

10   Helpful Therapies: Treatment Options to Consider   *149*

Appendices

A   Recommended Reading   *159*

B   Glossary   *163*

    References   *169*

    Index   *175*

Foreword

For many years, radiologists have treated patients with TMJ disorder based on X rays of their temporomandibular joints. Such treatment frequently meant surgery on the temporomandibular joint—unfortunately with varied and sometimes unsatisfactory results. As a radiologist I have seen the effects of some of these treatments. We are now finding that TMJ symptoms can originate away from the joint and therefore need a treatment that takes into account the whole patient.

Dr. Uppgaard has developed, and describes in this book, a method of treating TMJ that works well without using surgery. He has combined experience from his years of practice with his knowledge of medicine, dentistry, and complementary treatments in a way that few have done. After providing details about the disorder and the various methods of treatment, Dr. Uppgaard invites you, the reader, to become part of the healing process, to become involved in a healthy lifestyle that will benefit your TMJ disorder as well as your total health. He also includes information about diseases and conditions (like fibromyalgia) that are frequently related to TMJ disorder yet are rarely talked about in conjunction with it.

We in the medical profession are beginning to better understand the connection between the mind and the body and how this connection relates to stress. As a person becomes mentally stressed he or she can often transfer that stress to the body. For people with TMJ disorder the joint itself is frequently the repository of stress. Dr. Uppgaard offers ways to handle stress that are healthful and not damaging to the body.

Dr. Uppgaard is to be commended for persisting in his quest for a nonsurgical treatment for TMJ disorder and then presenting his findings in a clear fashion for the benefit of many who felt their problems were unsolvable. I compliment him, and you, the reader, for looking toward alternate solutions for a difficult, but not insurmountable, problem.

—Jim W. Baltzell, M.D.

Acknowledgments

How fortunate we professionals are who have benefited from the vast body of knowledge provided by such scholars as Janet Travell, M.D., David Simons, M.D., Nathan Allen Shore, D.D.S, Hans Selye, M.D., and others. Dr. Travell is regarded as the pioneer in pain diagnosis and management. Her research on referred pain revolutionized how TMJ disorder patients are treated today in major health clinics. Dr. Simons, co-author of *Myofascial Pain and Dysfunction: The Trigger Point Manual* with Dr. Travell, has provided much new information to our current understanding of trigger points. Dr. Shore provided the foundation for our understanding of the complexities of TMJ disorder through his writings in the early '50s and his dental textbook published in 1959. Dr. Hans Selye has been acclaimed throughout the world by scientists, physicians, and psychologists for his brilliant exposition of the stress theory. In his book, *The Stress of Life*, he explains how to combat disease by strengthening the body's own defenses against stress.

It is impossible for me to acknowledge adequately the many colleagues as well as patients who have contributed information and/or extended encouragement over the years. I especially want to mention the following:

Jim Baltzell, M.D.	Robin McKenzie, P.T.
John Barnes, P.T.	Larry Meskin, D.D.S., M.S.D., Ph.D.
George Eversaul, Ph.D.	Dave Mitchell, D.D.S., Ph.D.

Wm. Farrar, D.D.S.   Parker Mahan, D.D.S., Ph.D.

Jim Fricton, D.D.S., M.S.   Ken Olson, Ph.D.

Larry Funt, D.D.S., M.S.D.   L. D. Panky, D.D.S., M.S.

Harold Gelb, D.M.D.   Bonnie Prudden, P.T.

Charles S. Greene, D.D.S.   Mariano Rocabado, P.T.

Kate Hathaway, Ph.D.   Wm. Solberg, D.D.S., M.S.

Clayton M. Ingham, D.D.S.   Terry Spahl, D.D.S.

Peter Jannetta, M.D.   Brendan Stack, D.D.S., M.S.

Errol Lader, D.D.S.   John Witzig, D.D.S.

Wm. McCarty Jr., D.M.D.

I wish to thank Barb, my wife, friend, and partner, whose encouragement, patience, devotion and skilled editing enabled me to complete this project. Thanks also to my daughters Patricia Uppgaard and Katy Flaherty for their support and enthusiasm; to Dene Carney for his technical advice and direction early in the game; and to Dave and Mary Kolesar for their early advice and support. A special thanks to Claire Nagel for her creative illustrations and copyediting. And lastly, my sincere thanks to Dr. Roland Kehr for his friendship and support throughout the years.

Barb and I would both like to express our sincere appreciation to Catharine Sutker, Kristin Beck, and everyone at New Harbinger Publications for their warmth, enthusiasm, and professionalism. To Farrin Jacobs, senior editor, we say, "Your skill, your good humor, plus your untiring, undaunted efforts to keep us on track made this entire project an unforgettable and wonderful experience."

Introduction

Liz, a twenty-year-old who was attending college a great distance from my office, called in and said she was experiencing extreme pain, mainly on the left side of her head. She felt that her jaw was out of alignment; it would lock at times so she could not open her mouth. She also felt some clicking in the jaw area. Liz was desperate for help. These problems were affecting her ability to stay in school.

Getting Liz into the office was a virtual impossibility; yet she needed help immediately. I decided to try to work with her over the phone. After she returned the medical/dental questionnaire I had sent her, we set up a phone appointment. During that conversation, we talked about her condition and the Total Wellness Program, just as though she was in the office for her comprehensive consultation. I prescribed exercises for her to do to ease the pain and we set up an appointment during her winter break from school. She never needed that appointment!

Liz was the inspiration for this book. From my experience with her, I concluded that information about TMJ disorder could be presented in language that people could understand. Making people aware of the problem and helping them participate in their healing is the way of the future. Allowing people to take charge of their wellness and have confidence in their treatment plan is powerful medicine!

Liz is not the only patient who has been able to consult with me and then go on to make lifestyle changes and get well. Hundreds of patients have followed in her footsteps. You may be able to do the same. If you are presently seeing a health care professional for your

TMJ disorder, this book will help you understand your problem and what you can do to participate more fully in your treatment plan. In this book you'll find everything that I teach my patients to help them get well, stay well, and take charge of their health. Keep in mind that the information presented here is not intended to supplant successful, ongoing treatments but rather to enhance them.

Temporomandibular joint disorder, or TMJ disorder, is a problem in the jaw and surrounding areas of the head and neck that causes pain, discomfort, and disability in millions of people each year. It is estimated that 20 percent of the population will, at some time, suffer from some form of TMJ disorder, and fully 5 percent are desperate to find help. These numbers are staggering. Many people suffer needlessly as they search in vain for relief from their pain. Experts don't know why yet, but almost twice as many women as men are affected by TMJ disorder. Many millions of dollars are spent each year on medications to relieve pain, on unnecessary and costly tests, and on treatments that don't work. Sometimes surgeries are performed that not only do not help, but often make the problem worse.

TMJ disorder has many names. You might have been told you have TMJ, TMJ syndrome, TMJ dysfunction, or temporomandibular disorder (TMD). For our purposes we will use the term *TMJ disorder* because it is the most common and recognizable term. Even though TMJ disorder stands for temporomandibular joint disorder, it implies that the pain and problems can be in the jaw joint or in the muscles surrounding the joint, or both. TMJ is not just one disorder, but may be several conditions that affect, in addition to the jaw joint, the muscles surrounding the jaw as well. The Total Wellness Program as outlined in part 1 will help you manage your pain and provide you with insight into your particular condition.

Recent scientific research has provided new insights into TMJ disorder, especially in two important areas. One area that has been studied for many years, but doesn't get the attention it deserves, is whiplash injury resulting from motor vehicle accidents (MVAs). Since there are approximately 3.65 million whiplash injuries in the United States reported each year, the number of injured people is significant. Studies now confirm that between 87 and 97 percent of whiplash injuries from MVAs involve the jaw joint, as well as the neck (Garcia and Arrington 1996, 233). The jaw injury is called *mandibular whiplash,* just as the neck injury is called *cervical whiplash.* Often the injury to the temporomandibular joint is overlooked. A greater awareness of, and treatment for, mandibular whiplash among professionals who treat whiplash victims will result in a greater success rate in the future. See chapter 7 for more information about whiplash and TMJ disorder.

The other important area is the medical research currently being done on fibromyalgia. The American Medical Association recognized fibromyalgia as a syndrome in 1987. In the past this syndrome has been called fibrositis, myofascitis, myofibrositis, myogelosis, or myalgia (Fricton, Kroening, and Hathaway 1988, 67) and shares many symptoms with TMJ. Fibromyalgia research has provided a breakthrough in understanding TMJ disorder. In a number of cases the two disorders coexist. TMJ and fibromyalgia are very different disorders, however. Chapter 8 goes into the connection between them in detail.

With all of this new information emerging, you now will be able to better understand TMJ disorder and can become more proactive in your treatment and prevention of it. This book offers simple, conservative, and cost-effective steps that you can take to relieve pain, get well, and stay well. Once you have the information you need to help you understand your problem and the tools to work with at home to develop your own wellness plan, you'll be on your way to taking control of your TMJ. That's what this book is all about.

The Story behind the Program

Health care is changing dramatically in this country. Universal care is not a reality. Care is costly and often not available to the average citizen. As a result, there is much more emphasis on helping people to stay well, preventing disease, and most importantly, helping people participate in treatment decisions and options with their health care professionals.

Because my practice is in a rural area where patients have to travel great distances to receive services from specialized clinics, I decided to develop treatment plans and procedures involving active patient participation and education. The result has been highly successful, cost-effective, and conservative treatment for people suffering from TMJ disorders.

I stress the Total Wellness Program with all of my patients. When they recognize the importance of each step and the relationship between them, they heal much faster and stay well. The Program is not a magic formula that I dreamed up on my own; it evolved from years of studying successful techniques and treatment plans from the finest specialists and clinics in the United States. Of particular note is the University of Minnesota TMJ and Craniofacial Pain Clinic. Their multidisciplinary approach to the treatment of TMJ disorder is the foundation for everything I do in my practice.

When I began to recognize that a problem for many of my patients was the prohibitive distance from home to specialized clinics dealing with TMJ disorder, it became clear to me that the patients and I had to work on their TMJ-related problems together. I suspected that there was a way to guide my patients to heal themselves. My success with Liz gave me proof of that; so I began to dedicate myself to the task. My search for answers led me to Drs. David Simons and Janet Travell on the West Coast, and Drs. Harold Gelb, Larry Funt, and others on the East Coast. You will find information from these experts in this book, and I am grateful to all of them for their research, teachings, and perspectives.

The Total Wellness Program has been successful in hundreds of cases. I know this because I took the time to follow up and talk with these patients myself. If a patient does not show significant progress within a few weeks, I consider a referral to a specialist if this seems appropriate. Since I published a ten-year outcome-based study of 382 patients in 1992, I have continued to follow up with all patients who complete treatment. The responses are positive and gratifying:

- None of the patients has ever been referred for surgery.

- Most patients got well and remained well because they stuck with the Program.

- A few reported that they started to have problems and then remembered what they needed to do and got back on the Program.

- A few reported that it took longer than they expected, but eventually they were successful.

- Some returned to my office briefly if they regressed or were experiencing a stressful situation.

Although the follow-up with my patients was not a scientific study, the results gave me confidence that the Program can work for most people. Many physicians don't have time in their busy schedules to call their patients to see how they are doing, but I found this to be helpful not only for my study, but for my patient relationships as well. If you do choose to seek medical care for your TMJ disorder, having a doctor who listens to your concerns is an important part of successful treatment.

Charles S. Greene, D.D.S. (1992), Director of Orofacial Pain Studies at the University of Illinois College of Dentistry, agrees that communicating with patients is crucial for TMJ management. Because patients are often anxious about pain and its cause, open communication with their doctor or dentist can serve to soothe that anxiety. In other words, consulting an informed and understanding physician can be a helpful addition to your healing process.

Health care professionals must first be willing to believe their patients. When they do, a rapport develops that builds confidence between doctor and patient. When the patient is given the tools to become an active partner in the treatment plan, wonderful progress can be made. Confidence in your treatment plan is powerful medicine!

All too often, health care professionals focus on their own area of expertise rather than looking at the total patient. It is easy to see how this can happen when you consider the years of training necessary to become doctors or dentists and the emphasis placed on each person's chosen discipline. But progress is thwarted when the helping professions don't work together. How many dentists, for example, understand that most jaw problems are related to the muscles in the head, neck, shoulders, and total body? How many understand trigger points and referred pain? How many know how to properly construct a splint so it helps the patient, rather than making the problem worse? How many give unnecessary medications because they don't know what else to do? How many give up and send the patients away because they don't understand the total problem?

That is why it is so vitally important for you to understand the principles behind the Total Wellness Program and incorporate them into your daily life. No matter who you are seeing: doctor, dentist, physical therapist, specialist of any kind, the Program will help facilitate your healing. There is nothing invasive or irreversible in the Program. There is nothing that will make you feel worse. It won't even cost you any money, and you might be amazed at how good you will feel all over.

Let me tell you about my daughter Katy. When she was a new mother of twins, she developed a problem with carpal tunnel involving both wrists and fingers. She had surgery on the right wrist and was considering it for the other one. Meanwhile, she began to experience pain in her jaw and a recurrence of pain in the wrist that had been operated on. Naturally she came to her dad for help. We went over everything in the Total Wellness Program together and found that her posture was absolutely terrible; she was, after all, carrying around those two heavy babies. I gave her exercises to do for her jaw as well as for her total body. She did not require a splint. Katy's pain in her jaw went away in a few weeks, and so did the carpal tunnel pain. The twins are now fifteen years old, and Katy continues to follow the Program. If she slumps back into her old habits she knows what to do. She never required further treatment for either her TMJ disorder or her carpal tunnel syndrome.

You may have wondered what the *"and Related Disorders"* means in the title of this book. Katy's problem is an example of that. Poor posture and stressed muscles account for a huge percentage of the pain people experience in their everyday lives. The exercises in the Total Wellness Program can help ease more than just your jaw pain. So take a deep breath and keep reading. You're on your way to healing yourself.

How to Use This Book

This book is divided into two parts: "Your Total Wellness Program" and "Other Considerations in Taking Control of TMJ." Work through part 1 from beginning to end, filling in the charts and answering questionnaires as necessary. Use part 2 to help gather more information about the condition itself and the treatment opportunities available to you. The six steps to recovery in part 1 will be effective and helpful to you only if you treat them as a whole. You must work on all six areas together; make changes in all of them and give the plan some time to work. This is particularly true in breaking old habits that are keeping you from getting well and free of pain. Don't give up before you give yourself a chance to heal.

Remember that each person is unique. Just one event, accident, or faulty habit can set off problems throughout your entire body. Knowledge is power, and you are taking steps to gain the power to become a key player on your health care team. The intent of this book is to empower you to participate with your health care professionals in making the important decisions regarding your health. In order to do this you need to have the most accurate information available about TMJ disorder and possible treatment options. You need to determine what you can do to help yourself feel better. This involves carefully going over each chapter. Make necessary changes in your daily life, work, posture, and general habits. When you begin to do the prescribed exercises, you'll begin to feel better almost immediately.

You will find that my Program does not involve medications, surgery, injections, or X rays. The keys to success are in understanding the problem, having confidence in yourself, and faithfully following the Total Wellness Program. I have seen the Program work with hundreds of my patients and I have confidence that you, too, can achieve lifelong health and wellness.

Part I

Your Total Wellness Program

1

Understand the Problem

Are you one of the several million people who have pain in and around the jaw? Do you often get headaches for no apparent reason? Do you have difficulty opening and closing your mouth? Do you experience clicking or grating when you open or close your mouth? Does your jaw sometimes lock? Have you ever had pain in a perfectly healthy tooth? Do you clench and grind your teeth at night? Do you have tired or sore jaws when you wake up in the morning? Do you have difficulty hearing? Do you have ringing in your ears, pressure behind your eyes, or tearing for no apparent reason? Do you experience sinus pain?

If you answered Yes to any of these questions, you may have a TMJ disorder. In fact, you can just about count on it. Chances are you've already seen one or two health care professionals about your problem, but it hasn't gone away. You may have been given medications to relieve the pain—and that hasn't worked. You need some answers!

This chapter will give you the background and answers you need. In it, you'll find checklists, questions about your health history, a visual exam, and information about pain patterns. If you conclude that you may have a TMJ disorder, but don't feel that you can go through the Total Wellness Program on your own, you may want to search out a health care professional who can help you with your particular problem if you haven't done so already. There are many qualified professionals from different disciplines who can help you. See chapter 10 for some of the options in addition to those of your dentist and physician.

Mary, a thirty-year-old account executive with an advertising agency, worked long hours, traveled frequently, entertained business clients, and gave presentations often. She was also very active and enjoyed a variety of sports. Mary rarely went to the doctor, even though she frequently had headaches. She attributed her headaches mainly to stress. She also experienced stiffness in her neck. Her ears and jaw would often be sore if she spoke too much in one day or laughed a lot. Sometimes she could hear a clicking sound in her jaw. Mary ignored most of these discomforts.

In February, Mary was in a car accident. A driver ran a stop sign and hit her broadside. Mary did not seek treatment at the time; she regarded the accident as an inconvenience to her. As if Mary didn't have enough stress in her life, she was also planning for her wedding in the fall.

In April she received a notice for her regular dental checkup and she made the appointment. She had noticed that her teeth were not closing properly and she planned on asking her dentist about the "crooked bite." The dentist suspected TMJ disorder, but did not feel qualified to help Mary with the problem. He referred her to a specialist, who ordered X rays of Mary's jaw. The specialist recommended surgery to Mary to correct the jaw alignment and advised her that if proper action was not taken, she might not have a functioning jaw in the future.

Mary decided to get a second opinion and was referred to my office. I suggested a nonsurgical alternative for the problem. A splint was made for the lower teeth and I prescribed exercises. Mary had three or four appointments with me over a year and a half, and slowly the teeth aligned themselves again. The clicking stopped. Headaches still occur, but Mary recognizes their possible source and she practices self-help relaxation strategies. Most importantly, Mary avoided unnecessary surgery. "An unusual case?" Not at all. Why was Mary successful with her treatment plan?

- She understood how her jaw functions and learned that her jaw problems involved her total body.

- She got into the habit of doing jaw exercises and making postural changes.

- She gave up some harmful habits like clenching her teeth and chewing gum.

- She made lifestyle changes involving nutrition and exercise.

Everything that Mary learned is contained in this book. But none of it would have worked for her if she hadn't first made the effort to understand the problem. Understanding TMJ disorder is not an easy task. There are many big and complicated words. Some words can be simplified, others can't; but don't be discouraged. By working through this chapter you will come to understand the causes of your TMJ disorder and what to do about them. There is much that you can do for yourself once you have this information.

What Are the Temporomandibular Joints?

The *temporomandibular joints* are complex hinges that connect the lower jaw, or *mandible*, to the skull. They are made up of bones, ligaments, muscles, cartilage, and fascia. You have one on each side of your jaw. The joints move the jaw during chewing, speaking, swallowing, and so on. Place your fingertips against your face in front of your ears and move your jaw up and down; you can feel the temporomandibular joints. You use these hinges hundreds of times every day, even when you sleep.

The rounded ends at the top on each side of the mandible are called *condyles* (see figure 1.1). The condyles glide forward as the jaw opens. They slide back to their original position when you close your mouth. To keep this motion smooth, a soft *disc* lies between the condyle and the upper jaw, or *temporal bone*; this disc absorbs shocks to the temporomandibular joint from chewing and other movements. Because these joints are flexible, the jaw can move up and down and side to side, enabling you to talk, chew, and yawn.

Figure 1.2 shows the many muscles involved with the temporomandibular joint. When the jaw is not functioning properly, muscles begin to hold a tense, unnatural position. Muscle spasms occur, and before long the tension travels by chain reaction throughout the body. While an injured limb can be rested, it is impossible to leave the jaw joint inactive. That is why so many millions of people have problems—from very simple to extremely complex—in the temporomandibular joints.

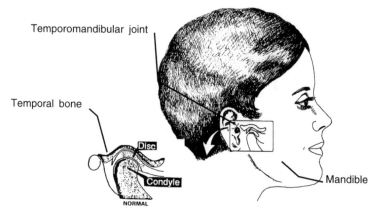

Temporomandibular joint

Temporal bone

Disc

Condyle

NORMAL

Mandible

Figure 1.1. Temporomandibular Joint

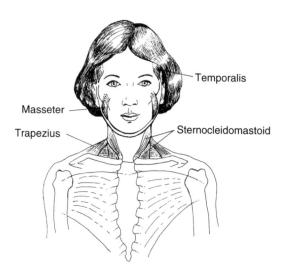

Temporalis

Masseter

Trapezius

Sternocleidomastoid

Figure 1.2. Muscles Related to Stress and TMJ Disorder

In addition to the bone, muscles, ligaments, and cartilage that make up the temporomandibular joint, many nerves and tiny blood vessels travel through the area (see figure 1.3). Any disruption of this flow can cause severe pain and discomfort.

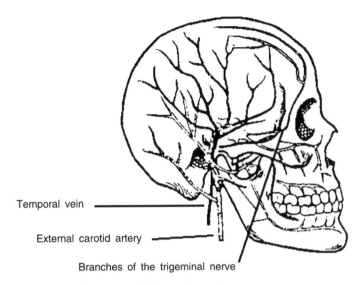

Temporal vein ────────────────

External carotid artery ──────

Branches of the trigeminal nerve

Figure 1.3. Nerves and Blood Vessels

What Is Temporomandibular Joint Disorder?

According to The National Institute of Dental Research, there is actually more than one type of TMJ disorder. They fall into three main categories:

- *Myofascial pain* (the most common form)—discomfort or pain in the muscles that control the jaw as well as the neck and shoulder muscles

- *Internal derangement of the joint*—a dislocated jaw or displaced disc, or injury to the condyle (see figure 1.5)

- *Degenerative joint disease*—for example, osteoarthritis or rheumatoid arthritis in the jaw joint.

You could have more than one of these conditions at the same time. I find that most of my patients with TMJ disorder have both myofascial pain and internal derangement. In addition, it should be noted that when a person has a coexisting systemic condition—such as fibromyalgia—with overlapping symptoms, the diagnosis and treatment become much more difficult.

Since myofascial pain is by far the most common form of TMJ disorder, that is the main area of focus in this book.

Myofascial Pain

In order to truly understand your TMJ Disorder, you must understand what myofascial pain means, what fascia is and how it affects your total well-being. Let's start with fascia:

What Is Fascia?

Fascia is the connective tissue found everywhere in your body that holds all of your organs in place. It joins every part of the body with every other part (Butler 1996). Fascia surrounds and invades every tissue and organ—including nerves, blood vessels, muscle, and bone—all the way down to the cellular level.

John Barnes, a physical therapist and founder of *Myofascial Release*, a gentle treatment for muscles in spasm, designed Fascia Man for teaching purposes. If you look at Fascia Man (figure 1.4), you will see that the majority of the fascia of the body goes vertically, from head to toe. However, there are four other planes of fascia, all inter-connected, that crisscross the body in a weblike manner. They are called transverse planes. Why is this important for you to know? According to Barnes (1990, 18),

> When fascia malfunctions due to injury, illness, surgery, poor posture or inflammation, it becomes tight and binds down, resulting in abnormal pressure on nerves, muscles, bones or organs of the body. This excessive pressure can produce pain, headaches, TMJ Dysfunction and restriction of motion.
>
> Why should we be concerned about fascia in the legs or back? Because, if injury occurs in one part of the body, the binding down can create pain and malfunction throughout the body! This is because the fascia of the body is all interconnected, and a restriction in one region can put a "drag" on the fascia in any other direction.

Barnes (1995) describes the following other important factors concerning fascia:

- Fascia supports and stabilizes, thus enhancing the postural balance of the body.

- It is vitally involved in all acts of motion and acts as a shock absorber.

- It aids in circulation of the blood and lymphatic fluids.

- It is a major area of inflammatory processes; that is, it is involved when there is any tissue irritation, injury, or infection, characterized by pain, redness, localized fever, or swelling.

- The central nervous system is surrounded by fascial tissue, which attaches to the inside of the cranium. Dysfunction in these tissues can have a profound and widespread neurological effect.

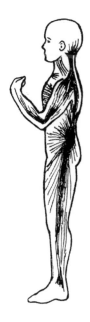

Figure 1.4. Fascia Man

Reprinted with permission of John Barnes, P.T.

What Does Myofascia Mean?

There are different types of connective tissue, or fascia. The one we are concerned with is called *myofascia*. "Myo" means muscle; so this type of fascia is involved with the muscles of the body. Butler (1996, 4) writes,

Certain types of fascia known as myofascia permeate through muscle, first wrapping individual muscle fibers, then bundles of muscle fibers, then bundles of bundles, and finally the entire muscle structure. Where the muscle fibers end, the myofascia that has been wrapping all of those fibers continues, becoming the tendon. Tendon actually blends into bone, becoming part of it. With a tensile strength greater than that of steel, fascia is an extremely durable component of the body.

What Is Myofascial Pain?

Myofascial pain, then, is pain resulting from changes in the fascial system of your body and involves the muscles. In TMJ disorder, professionals tend to look primarily at the muscles of the upper body and head. While this is the main site of pain, the rest of the body should not be overlooked. Myofascial pain occurs throughout the body and affects how healing takes place. The Total Wellness Program looks at the body from head to toe, which is the reason, I believe, the Program has been so successful.

Internal Derangement

If the disc is pushed forward (as in figure 1.5) the joint will not work properly, and TMJ problems result. The diagnosis is *internal derangement.*

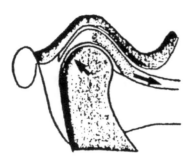
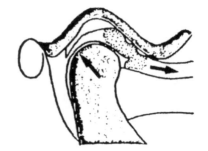

a. Slight displacement   b. Advanced displacement

Figure 1.5. Internal Derangement

What Causes TMJ Disorders?

Medical and dental communities are divided over what causes TMJ disorder and just as divided on what to do about it. When a jaw joint is not working properly, and pain and disability occur, an attempt is always made to identify a cause. However, trying to pinpoint a cause is frequently not fruitful for the following reasons (Greene 1992, 43):

- Patients often have more than one problem at the same time that may or may not be related. For example, a patient may have recurring headaches and a benign TMJ problem, such as painless clicking.

- Jaw pain can be referred from other areas, such as the sinuses, or dental conditions.

- TMJ symptoms can be part of a systemic problem, such as fibromyalgia, rheumatoid arthritis, lupus, or others.

It is of the utmost importance to identify all the factors in your life that contribute to the problem, as well as the immediate event that set it off. If you look at causes and contributing factors together, you will get to the solution of the problem much faster.

Causes and contributing factors can be separated into general areas and include the following:

Dental

- Poor bite (malocclusion)

- Missing teeth that have not been replaced (resulting in jaw overclosure)

- Past dental surgery

- Any opening of the jaw for a prolonged period, even a big yawn

- Poorly fitting or worn-out dentures

Injuries

- Whiplash

- Traction appliances used in whiplash injuries which place undue stress on the jaw

- A blow to the head, face, or jaw (may be considered minor; may not be recent)

Habits

- Bad posture, such as slouching, holding the phone on your shoulder, sleeping on your stomach, sitting in poorly designed chairs, and so on

- Bad habits at work, particularly posture at the computer

- Oral habits such as pencil biting, gum chewing, or clenching (bruxing) when under stress

- Childhood habits such as thumbsucking or deviant swallowing habits

- Poor diet or eating habits

- Activities, such as heavy lifting, that strain the neck or the back

Adverse social situations that cause undue stress

- Bad home situation

- Recent stressful events

- Financial worries

- Difficulties at work

- Litigation

- Life changes, such as divorce or death of a loved one

Emotional

- Depression (acute or chronic)

- Anger

- Anxiety

- Frustration

- Unrelieved stress

- Fear

TMJ disorder can start at an early age and get progressively worse. Two outstanding dentists, Drs. Lawrence Funt and Brendan Stack, published a study of many patients from ages four to seventy.

The study showed how symptoms of TMJ disorder increase in both number, as well as severity, as you get older. A version of their *F-S Index of the Craniomandibular Pain Syndrome* appears in figure 1.6.

To read the *F-S Index*, look for your age group at the bottom. Are you having any of the symptoms that appear to the left of the bar in your age category? There will of course be variations from person to person. Check other age categories. Did you have similar symptoms when you were younger? By looking at older ages you will learn what could happen as you age unless you take control of the problem.

What Are the Most Common Symptoms of TMJ Disorder?

Symptoms of TMJ disorder can occur around the jaw, around the head, and throughout the total body and will vary from person to person. Later in this chapter you will be asked to fill out a checklist of your own symptoms.

Around the Jaw

- Clicking, grating, or popping in the jaw

- Pain in and around the jaw

- Clenching and grinding while you sleep or during the day

- Difficulty opening your mouth

- Difficulty closing your mouth

- Jaw locks open or shut

- Pain in the teeth

- Tired or sore jaw when you wake up

- Jaw deviates on opening and closing

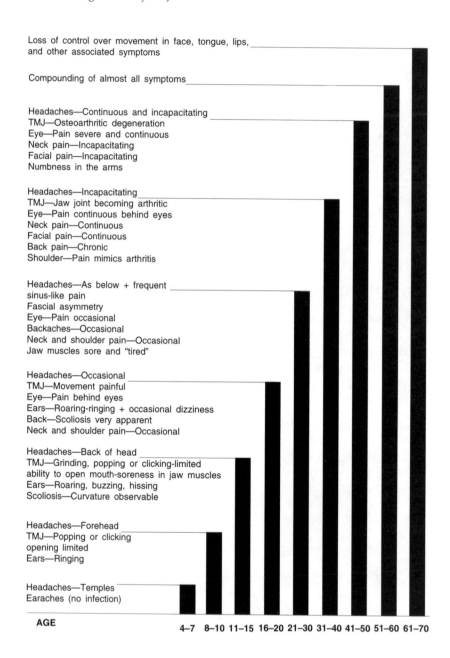

Loss of control over movement in face, tongue, lips, and other associated symptoms

Compounding of almost all symptoms

Headaches—Continuous and incapacitating
TMJ—Osteoarthritic degeneration
Eye—Pain severe and continuous
Neck pain—Incapacitating
Facial pain—Incapacitating
Numbness in the arms

Headaches—Incapacitating
TMJ—Jaw joint becoming arthritic
Eye—Pain continuous behind eyes
Neck pain—Continuous
Facial pain—Continuous
Back pain—Chronic
Shoulder—Pain mimics arthritis

Headaches—As below + frequent
sinus-like pain
Fascial asymmetry
Eye—Pain occasional
Backaches—Occasional
Neck and shoulder pain—Occasional
Jaw muscles sore and "tired"

Headaches—Occasional
TMJ—Movement painful
Eye—Pain behind eyes
Ears—Roaring-ringing + occasional dizziness
Back—Scoliosis very apparent
Neck and shoulder pain—Occasional

Headaches—Back of head
TMJ—Grinding, popping or clicking-limited
ability to open mouth-soreness in jaw muscles
Ears—Roaring, buzzing, hissing
Scoliosis—Curvature observable

Headaches—Forehead
TMJ—Popping or clicking
opening limited
Ears—Ringing

Headaches—Temples
Earaches (no infection)

AGE

4–7   8–10 11–15 16–20 21–30 31–40 41–50 51–60 61–70

Figure 1.6. The F-S Index* of the Craniomandibular Pain Syndrome

---

*   Reprinted with permission of contributing authors of *The Clinical Management of Head, Neck and Jaw Dysfunction* as published by W. B. Saunders Company, December 1997. Edited as an aid to lay persons.

Clicking

Most people with TMJ disorder experience either clicking or grating noises in the jaw joint. Sometimes it causes pain or discomfort. Many of my patients are anxious or concerned about the noise. Therefore, I go over the diagram in figure 1.7 with them so they understand what is taking place in the jaw joint when they open and close the jaw. The diagram was created by Drs. Farrar, McCarty, and Witzig. It shows the condyle in a displaced starting position (A), behind the disc. When diagnosing internal derangement, physicians listen for a click as the mouth opens and closes. The opening click takes place from B to C, and the closing click takes place from F to A. The dotted lines indicate the displaced starting position of the condyle. When the disc is pushed forward, the condyle has to override the thickness of the disc, which results in a click. It can click as the jaw opens or as the jaw closes and the condyle returns to its displaced position behind the disc.

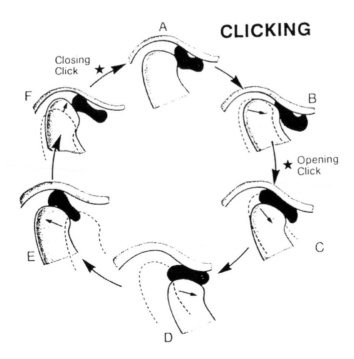

Figure 1.7. Clicking

Around the Head

- Difficulty swallowing
- Muscle soreness or spasms around the head or neck
- Ringing in the ears
- Difficulty hearing
- Frequent earaches with no infection present
- Headaches of all kinds
- Sinus pains
- Pressure behind the eyes
- Tearing for no reason

Throughout the Total Body

- Muscle spasms in the neck, shoulders, back, arms, or legs
- Numbness in arms or fingers
- Dizziness
- Backaches
- Cold hands and feet
- Arthritis

In addition, patients with TMJ disorder frequently report difficulty sleeping, fatigue, nervousness, anger, and depression. Is it any wonder that professionals have difficulty diagnosing this elusive problem? Except for the symptoms around the jaw, the other symptoms could be caused by any number of diseases. Often other diseases are checked out and medications given to try to alleviate the pain and discomfort before a TMJ disorder is diagnosed.

Do You Have a TMJ Disorder?

The following checklists and questionnaires will help you assess your symptoms, health history, and habits to determine the probability of a TMJ disorder. Go over each section carefully, and a pattern will develop that reflects your own particular life experiences.

Symptoms Checklist

Do you have any of the following symptoms? Put a checkmark next to the symptoms that apply to you.

Area 1: Around the Jaw

_____ Clicking, grating, or popping in the jaw joint

_____ Pain in and/or around the jaw

_____ Clenching or grinding teeth while you sleep or during the day

_____ Difficulty opening your mouth

_____ Difficulty closing your mouth

_____ Jaw locks open or shut

_____ Pain in the teeth

_____ Tired or sore jaw when you wake up

_____ Jaw deviates on opening and closing

Area 2: Around the Head

_____ Difficulty swallowing

_____ Muscle soreness or spasms around the head and neck

_____ Ringing in the ears

_____ Difficulty hearing

_____ Frequent earaches with no infection present

_____ Headaches of all kinds

_____ Sinus pain

_____ Pressure behind the eyes

_____ Tearing for no reason

Area 3: Throughout the Body

_____ Muscle spasms in the neck, shoulder, back, arms, or legs

_____ Numbness in arms or fingers

_____ Dizziness

_____ Backaches

_____ Difficulty sleeping

_____ Fatigue, nervousness, anger, or depression

_____ Arthritis

Conclusion

If you have one or more symptoms from Area 1, in addition to any symptoms from either Area 2 or Area 3, you should suspect a TMJ disorder.

Coexisting Condition

Now that you've figured out that you may have a TMJ disorder, it's time to look deeper into your condition. Thanks to Dr. Edward Wright et al. (1997), the following questions are designed to help identify a possible coexisting rheumatic condition:

1. Do you have muscle tenderness other than in your head and neck?

   _____ Yes _____ No

2. Do you have joint tenderness other than in your jaw joint?

   _____ Yes _____ No

3. Do you have morning stiffness other than in the jaw?

   _____ Yes _____ No

4. Do you have muscle tenderness other than in your head or neck more than 50 percent of the time?

   _____ Yes _____ No

5. Do you have joint tenderness other than in your jaw joint more than 50 percent of the time?

   _____ Yes _____ No

6. Over the past year, have you had recurrent swelling of joints other than in your temporomandibular joints?

_____ Yes _____ No

Conclusion

If you answered Yes to any of these questions you need to consult a doctor familiar with rheumatic disorders (see chapter 8), in addition to a dentist skilled in the diagnosis and treatment of TMJ disorder.

Health History

Think carefully about your past history from birth to present. There are factors that make you more susceptible to TMJ disorders. Perhaps you were born with a jaw malformation, however slight. You may have had an early accident or blow to the head. You might have been a thumb sucker. Sometimes an early illness weakens the immune system. Allergies are frequently the culprit. We call these *predisposing factors*. They happened long ago and set you up for future problems.

Sometimes an unusual event that is abrupt or unexpected occurs during your lifetime and sets off your TMJ disorder. This could be a blow to the head, an auto accident, even a yawn, surgery, or certain medications. We call these *precipitating factors*.

After you have the start of a TMJ disorder, you can cause it to continue indefinitely by faulty habits, such as gum chewing, jaw clenching, poor posture, lack of proper exercise, or improper diet. We call these *perpetuating factors* because they tend to prolong the existence of the problem.

Check off anything that you are aware of in your history that could relate to having a TMJ disorder. Please understand this is not a comprehensive medical history. The purpose is to make you aware of events in your life that might be contributing to the problem that you have today.

Predisposing Factors

_____ Bodily abnormality such as a short leg

_____ Early accident

_____ Jaw abnormality

_____ Thumb sucking

_____ Blow to the head

_____ Severe illness

_____ Allergies

Precipitating Factors

_____ Blow to the head

_____ Auto accident

_____ Surgery

_____ Medications

_____ Yawn or opening your mouth unusually wide

Perpetuating Factors

Mechanical stresses

_____ Occlusal habits:

    _____ Gum chewing

    _____ Jaw clenching

    _____ Pencil biting

_____ Postural habits at work:

    _____ Phone on shoulder

    _____ Sitting wrong at the computer

    _____ Lifting improperly

_____ Postural habits at home:

    _____ Slouching on the couch

    _____ Improper bending

    _____ Phone on shoulder

_____ Postural habits anytime:

    _____ Head protruded

    _____ Slouching while walking

    _____ Crossing one leg over another while sitting

    _____ Sitting in ill-fitting furniture, such as a seat too deep or chair arms too high

    _____ Prolonged immobility

_____ Abuse of muscles:

    _____ Overstressing muscles in exercise

    _____ Constricting pressure on muscles, such as wearing clothing that is too tight, or carrying a heavy shoulder bag

Nutritional inadequacies (Refer to chapter 6)

    _____ Low levels of B_1, B_6, B_{12}, and folic acid

    _____ Vitamin C deficiency

    _____ Calcium, potassium, and iron deficiencies

    _____ Poor diet in general

Psychological stresses

    _____ Depression

    _____ Tension caused by anxiety

    _____ Unrelieved stress

Other

    _____ Chronic infection due to viral/bacterial disease

    _____ Impaired sleep

Conclusion

If you answered Yes to any of these questions and are experiencing pain, you should suspect a TMJ disorder. Read on!

Visual Exam

Do this exam while looking in the mirror.

1. Open and close your mouth. Does your jaw deviate to the right, left, or to both sides when you open wide?

    ____ Yes ____ No

2. Are there any noises from the jaw joint?

    ____ Yes ____ No

3. Open your mouth as wide as you can (without pain). Can you fit three fingers in when you open? (See figure 1.8.)

    ____ Yes ____ No

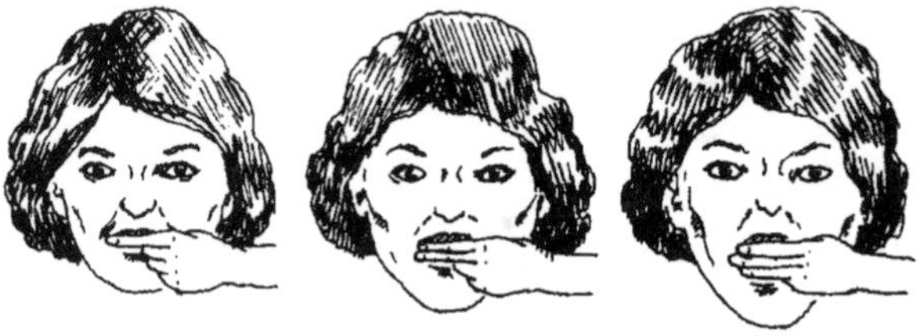

Figure 1.8.

Conclusion

If you answered Yes to 1 and 2 and No to 3 you may confirm your suspicions of having a TMJ disorder.

Feature Imbalance

As you continue to look in the mirror, look for *feature imbalance*. (See figure 1.9.) According to Gelb (1980):

> This is one of the most definitive indications of a jaw imbalance. Often by just looking at a person's face, you can tell on which side the jaw is unbalanced, as well as on which side the pain is developing.
>
> Stand in front of a full-length mirror so that you can check for imbalances down the whole body. Look at your face. Is one eye higher or larger than the other?

Are your lips turned up on the side of the higher eye? Is the ear on that higher side higher than the other ear?

If your answer to these questions was Yes, you probably have a jaw imbalance on the side of your face where the features are higher.

If you continue down the body, you'll find that the level of the shoulders, breasts and hips are lower on the side where the facial features are higher. The leg on this side is usually shorter than the other, too.

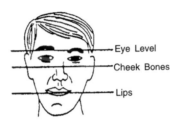

Figure 1.9.

Pain Patterns around the Head and Neck

Check for pain patterns around your head and neck. You can check most of these yourself by pressing firmly with one or two fingers.

_____ Above your ear

_____ In front of your ear

_____ In your ear

_____ In the cheek muscle that tightens up when you clench your teeth

_____ In the muscles under the ear

_____ In the shoulder muscles

_____ In the muscles behind the neck

Conclusion

Pain patterns in the muscles around the head and neck are common indicators of a TMJ disorder. If you have answered Yes to any question in this section you should suspect TMJ disorder.

Pain Patterns throughout the Body

In figure 1.10 place an X on all areas of the body where you experience pain most of the time. This includes hands, feet, wrists, toes, and so on. Chapter 3 goes into detail on how muscles in other parts of the body refer pain to the jaws and head. All you need to know is that poor posture and faulty habits result in improper body alignment, which causes a host of problems throughout the entire body.

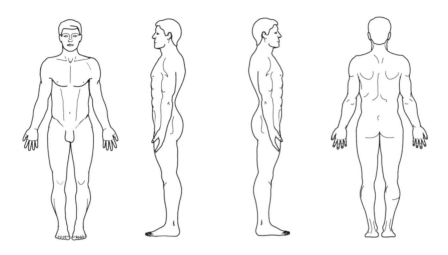

Figure 1.10. Pain Patterns throughout the Body

Conclusion

If you have marked areas of your body where you have pain and have answered Yes to any of the other questions in this chapter you can confirm your TMJ disorder.

You have worked hard on this chapter, and it was not easy reading. You have completed your personal inventory, have a basic understanding of TMJ disorder, and know whether or not you may be a victim. You are ready to learn what you can do to feel better and to participate in your treatment program. I encourage you to go through these next chapters carefully, because in them you will find solutions to many of your health problems.

2

Exercises to Improve Jaw Functioning

When pain is present in the jaw area, there are exercises that can be done specifically to help relieve the pain and prevent its recurrence. These exercises, developed by Mariano Rocabado, P.T., recognized worldwide for his leadership in managing TMJ disorder, are an important part of the Total Wellness Program. The first five exercises are designed to improve jaw functioning. The next four exercises are designed to correct postural concerns of the head and neck. I advise making the exercises in this chapter a daily routine. They will teach you to avoid clenching, help you stretch your jaw and neck muscles, and correct muscular imbalance.

Because clenching is at the root of most jaw problems, in addition to doing these exercises you must learn to be aware of when you're clenching. You tend to clench when you're busy, when you're concentrating on something, or when you are stressed. Some people clench or grind their teeth as they sleep, and wake up in the morning with sore jaws. Breaking the habit of clenching, then, is the most important task in your six steps to recovery.

Sometimes a splint, or night-guard, is needed to prevent clenching at night. However, if you break the habit during the day, this can carry over to your nighttime habits as well. At least try it for a while before you resort to a night-guard. If you are advised to have a night-guard, read chapter 9, which gives information about splints.

Chapter 6 provides total body exercises that are important to your physical well-being.

Cheryl is a busy woman. Not only is she a wife and mother of two, but she also runs an educational consulting business, is active in civic affairs, and is on the board of directors of the local hospital. A perfectionist in all she does, she does it all well. Cheryl does not have time to be sick, and usually enjoys very good health. Here is what she said about her TMJ disorder:

> I first met Dr. Bob several years ago on referral from my dentist to help me control clenching. This behavior had caused facial pain, bite alignment problems, and tooth problems. Dr. Bob suggested some jaw exercises. I was amazed at the results of just doing these simple exercises. They solved my problem. I learned to relax my jaw at tense times, and eventually it became a positive habit. He also identified some pain points, he calls them trigger points, in my temple, neck, shoulders, and back; but the jaw was my primary concern and focus at that time.
>
> A few years later I experienced severe facial pain after I broke a tooth, and those pain points were again brought to my attention by Dr. Bob. The broken tooth caused a series of gum, root, and alignment complications, which all culminated in almost constant and uncontrollable facial, temple, sinus, and neck pain. He again found all of those sensitive spots in my temple, neck, shoulders, and back. The combination of applying pressure on these pain points and deep breathing began to ease the facial pain, and the pathways of referred pain began to make sense. When the tooth was successfully repaired, the pain ended, but the awareness of the referred pain made a lasting impression. I realized that the pain points were related to posture, muscle use, and probably complicated by my scoliosis. Periodically the facial pain will begin to recur, and I am able to control it by improving my posture, not sleeping on the affected side, exercising, massage, deep breathing and, of course, doing the jaw exercises.

Let's go through the exercises. They are designed specifically to improve the functioning of the jaw and teach postural awareness and correction. The goal is to gently bring the jaw into proper balance and to help the jaw muscles relax. The first six exercises can be done in any position and should not last for more than one minute each. Try to do the series six times daily.

Exercise 1: Avoiding Clenching

This is by far the most important exercise. I encourage you to practice it and make it part of your daily life.

Purpose

This exercise trains you to keep your jaw relaxed at all times, thus enabling the jaw to maintain a resting position and the muscles to totally relax.

Precautions

None.

The Exercise

1. Make a "cluck" sound with your tongue. The front third of your tongue should rest on the roof of your mouth.

2. Maintain this position using slight pressure. Do not allow the tongue to touch the teeth.

3. Keep your lips together.

4. Your teeth should be slightly apart and your lower jaw should be completely relaxed.

5. Breathe through your nose. Breathe deeply, from the diaphragm rather than from the chest.

I recommend making this exercise a lifelong habit. Always remember:

- Lips together

- Teeth slightly apart

- Tongue resting on the roof of the mouth

- Lower jaw relaxed

Exercise 2: Stretching the Jaw and Increasing Range of Motion

Purpose

This exercise helps you to relax the opening muscles, stretch the closing muscles, and remediate limited jaw opening.

Precautions

Do not do this exercise if your jaw is acutely strained or if you experience grating, clicking, or popping.

The Exercise

Refer to figure 2.1 to see what this exercise should look like. Do the exercise for one to two minutes, twice a day. Use ice or moist heat, whichever feels comfortable to you, over the sore area of the muscle as you do this exercise.

1. Gradually increase your jaw opening by placing one knuckle or an object of equivalent size between the teeth.

2. Rest on knuckle or object for sixty seconds.

3. Increase to two knuckles and finally three, as you feel comfortable.

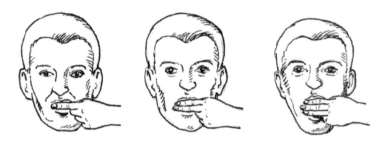

Figure 2.1. Stretching the Jaw

Exercise 3: Increasing Jaw Opening

Purpose

This exercise helps you to relax the closing muscles and strengthen the chewing muscles.

Precautions

Use gentle pressure only.

The Exercise

Refer to figure 2.2 to see what this exercise should look like. Do the exercise ten times, twice a day.

1. Make a fist and place it against your chin between the pointer finger and second fingers.

2. With your teeth slightly apart, gently push upward (figure 2.2a).

3. Open against this pressure to one finger width (figure 2.2b). Hold for a count of ten.

4. Remove fist from under jaw and close (figure 2.2c).

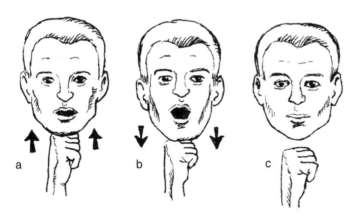

Figure 2.2. Increasing Jaw Opening

Exercise 4: Rhythmic Stabilization

Purpose

This exercise helps you to correct any muscular imbalance that may be present and promotes even force distribution between the temporomandibular joints. In other words, you will guide the jaw so that it does not deviate to either side on opening and closing in order to establish proper jaw opening and closing patterns.

Precautions

Do not use excessive force.

The Exercise

Do this exercise while sitting comfortably in front of a mirror. Refer to figure 2.3 to see what this exercise should look like.

1. Place your tongue in proper position with the front third of it resting on the roof of your mouth, not touching teeth (as in exercise 1).

2. Grasp your chin by placing your index fingers over your chin and your thumbs under your chin.

3. Open your jaw straight down to about two fingers width. Try not to deviate to one side. Apply gentle resistance as you open and close.

4. Apply gentle resistance as you move the lower jaw sideways, to the right, then to the left.

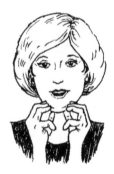

Figure 2.3. Rhythmic Stabilization

Exercise 5: Control TMJ Rotation

Purpose

This exercise teaches proper jaw motion.

Precautions

None.

The Exercise

1. Hold your tongue in correct position (as in exercise 1).

2. Place your index fingers over the temporomandibular joint (as in figure 2.4).

3. Open and close your mouth, stopping if you feel the condyle ("ball") of the joint move forward against your fingers. Do not allow your tongue to leave your palate.

Note: Chewing in this shortened range is often helpful.

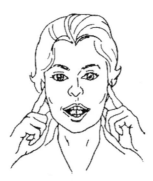

Figure 2.4. Controlling TMJ Rotation

Exercise 6: Head and Neck Stretch

This exercise should be done *only under the supervision of your doctor, dentist, physical therapist,* or other health care professional who understands your physical condition.

Purpose

This exercise helps you to gently stretch the muscles of the posterior and lateral neck and head areas. When the many muscles involved with TMJ disorder become tight or go into spasm, a gentle progressive stretching of the muscles is needed to alleviate the problem.

Precautions

This exercise should be performed gently. Overstretching may make the condition worse. A general rule is to stretch slightly further than the point where you feel a little tension.

The Exercise

Refer to figure 2.5 to see what this exercise should look like. Do this exercise twice daily, unless otherwise advised, gradually increasing the stretch. Hold for five seconds.

1. Gently grasp the left side of your head with your right hand while reaching behind your back with the other hand. Make sure your shoulders are straight and posture good. Aim your ear toward your armpit.

2. Tilt head down until a gentle stretch is felt. Hold for five seconds.

3. Repeat on the other side.

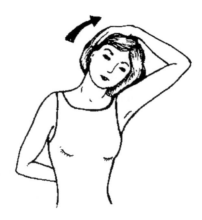

Figure 2.5. Head and Neck Stretch

Exercise 7: Improve Shoulder Posture

Purpose

This exercise stretches your chest muscles and improves lung capacity, helping you to stay more relaxed and keep your jaw in a healthy position.

Precautions

None.

The Exercise

At the same time as you are practicing exercise 1, pull your shoulder blades together and downward (figure 2.6).

Incorrect   Correct

Figure 2.6. Improve Shoulder Posture

Exercise 8: Stabilization Head Flexion

Purpose

This exercise stretches muscles in your back and neck.

Precautions

None.

The Exercise

1. Clasp hands firmly behind your neck (to stabilize neck).

2. Keep head straight, then nod your head forward.

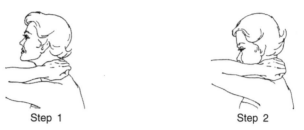

Step 1   Step 2

Figure 2.7. Stabilization Head Flexion

Exercise 9: Axial Extension of Neck

Purpose

This exercise will help you to get the feel of the proper position for your head.

Precautions

None.

The Exercise

1. Do these three motions at once, gently: nod your head, glide your neck backward, and stretch your head upward (figure 2.8).

2. Think of your chin being comfortably closer to your neck.

Incorrect   Correct

Figure 2.8. Axial Extension of Neck

Although the Rocabado exercises are extremely important in treating TMJ disorder, there is much more to learn about this area of the body. Especially important is the pain that comes from muscles, which is called referred pain from trigger points. Read on.

3

Treat Referred Pain from Trigger Points

Muscles are funny things. They can knot up on you sometimes, and cause a lot of pain. You know this if you've ever had a cramp in your leg, or charley horse. You had to stop doing what you were doing and rub the cramp until the muscle released. Well, muscles can play other tricks on you, too. Sometimes a muscle in one part of your body can cause pain in another part of your body. Most of the time you don't even realize that the culprit is a faraway muscle.

Peggy, a thirty-nine-year-old housewife, was in a lot of pain as a result of an automobile accident fifteen months earlier. She was referred to me by her family dentist. She had already been to see her family physician, an orthopedic surgeon, and a physical therapist for pain in her shoulder. Painkillers, muscle relaxants, and a neck brace were all ineffective.

When I asked her about her symptoms, Peggy reported fatigue, cold hands and feet, clenching, ringing in her ears, hearing loss, and frequent earaches. She also suffered occasionally from headaches, backaches, sinus problems, and numbness in her fingers. Her jaw often locked shut. She could only open her mouth to 27 millimeters (just over an inch), and even then there was pain and a grating noise in her jaw joint. (A 40-millimeter opening is considered normal.) Peggy also reported a tense neck, frustration, fear, mood swings, and anxiety. Her anxiety often caused her to bite her nails.

As I examined Peggy and pressed on specific muscles of the head, neck, and shoulders, she experienced intense pain. I discovered some hard little nodules in the muscles being pressed. Peggy, like most people, did not know that these painful areas in her neck and shoulders were related to her jaw pain and opening problems. Once I explained the connection and what she could do to avoid the problem, Peggy took charge of her healing by faithfully following the Total Wellness Program.

After only six days following her initial appointment, Peggy was feeling much better. She reported, "I feel pretty good. I can sleep at night, and my jaw doesn't lock. My husband can't believe what you have done." Eleven months later she reported that she was "doing great."

What Peggy was experiencing is called *referred pain from trigger points*. Once you understand this phenomenon and take action to change it, you'll find more relief from the pain of TMJ disorder.

Referred Pain and Trigger Points

Almost all TMJ disorder patients have *referred pain* from some muscle, if not many muscles, from head to toe. This is why it is important for you to understand what referred pain and trigger points are, and how they relate to you. The hard nodules in Peggy's muscles that were sensitive to touch are called *trigger points*. Pain is felt not only in these trigger points, but also in areas remote from the site of the trigger point. This is called *referred pain*.

Once you know which muscle is involved, if you press on the hard little knot or nodule there, you will most likely jump with pain. The trigger point, also called a *myofascial trigger point*, lies somewhere along the referring muscle, which is very tight. The muscle is usually described as "a taut band," and it feels sinewy because it has tightened up from overuse, trauma of some sort, poor posture, or other reasons. By eliminating the trigger point in the muscle, you also eliminate the pain in the faraway area.

The good news is that these pain patterns are predictable. Referred pain patterns from trigger points are the same for all people! In 1983, Drs. Janet Travell and David Simons published *Myofascial Pain and Dysfunction: The Trigger Point Manual*, in which they diagrammed and described these pain patterns. Their research has enabled health care professionals from many disciplines to track the pain patterns of their patients, help eliminate the pain, and prevent its recurrence. The patient provides the most valuable information for finding where the trigger point is located by describing the precise pattern of pain. The clinician will generally recognize the pattern of pain as characteristic of a particular muscle and will know where to look for the trigger point (or trigger points) responsible for at least some of the pain. After you read this chapter, you will be able to do this, too.

The most current comprehensive information available today on referred pain from trigger points comes from recent studies by David G. Simons, M.D. (1996; 1993). He has found not only that trigger points are a common cause of musculoskeletal (muscular) pain and dysfunction, but that there are certain clinical features common in most patients. According to Simons (1996, 98),

- There is usually a history of acute muscle overload or chronic abuse of the muscle.

- Spot tenderness involves a very tender and very small, nodular spot, which is found in a palpable band. [Tight muscle in spasm. One you can feel.] Sometimes a trigger point is located deep within the body, and the palpable band cannot be felt. Spot tenderness is the only clue.

- Pressure on the spot of tenderness causes the patient to physically react to the pain with a spontaneous exclamation or movement. This is called a Jump Sign, and [is] a significant clue that the patient has a trigger point in that muscle.

- An active trigger point (TrP) refers pain in a pattern characteristic of that muscle.

- Clinically, the patient is unable to produce normal strength in the affected muscle, especially when performing a common activity that uses the muscle.

- An active trigger point can recover spontaneously, may persist without progression or, with aggravating perpetuating factors, may develop additional trigger points (105).

- After an individual develops an active trigger point, especially in the absence of any perpetuating factor, continuing normal gentle daily activity and avoiding muscle overload often permit spontaneous regression from an active trigger point to a latent one in a few days to a few weeks (106). [It is still there, but it doesn't bother you.]

- The presence of perpetuating factors assures persistence of an active trigger point and sets the stage for the development of secondary trigger points, additional symptoms, and chronicity, with progressive functional disability and psychological distress. The presence of perpetuating factors is one of the most common, and often one of the most important, factors in the management of patients with chronic myofascial trigger points (1996, 106).

- Treatment is aimed at releasing the trigger points and restoring normal tension at resting muscle length. (Resting length may not change—tension does).

It is important to note that not all pain in your body comes from trigger points. Pain can result from other traumas, diseases, or illnesses. However, as far as TMJ disorder is concerned, Greene states that most modern authorities now regard TMJ problems as benign muscular conditions that can be treated and reversed by simple measures (1992). Long-term studies have shown that 80 to 90 percent of these patients can expect both good short-term results and little or no long-term problems after conservative therapy that reduces pain and restores normal muscle function. That is why it is so vitally important for you to understand the information in this section. It's not easy reading; but it is your key to getting well and staying well. Take your time, study each muscle group, and make note of muscles that are hurting you.

Pain Referral Patterns from Head, Neck, and Shoulder Muscles

This section details the major muscle groups that refer pain to the jaw area and will help you locate your trigger points. As you look at the drawings that go along with each muscle, press firmly on your own muscles and see if you can find any trigger points*. You will know when you hit one! Start at the top of a muscle and run your fingers along the muscle. You may find a hard little nodule or knot. If you press firmly on the knot and feel severe pain, you have likely found a trigger point. However, finding trigger points is only part of the solution. There are four steps to easing referred pain from trigger points.

1. Find the trigger point.

---

* Figures 3.1-3.8 reprinted with permission from Drs. Travell and Simons, authors of *Myofascial Pain and Dysfunction: The Trigger Point Manual* (Baltimore: Williams & Wilkens Co., 1983). Second edition available in 1999. Text and information provided by Starlanyl and Copeland, *Fibromyalgia and Chronic Myofascial Pain Syndrome*, (Oakland: New Harbinger Publications, 1996).

2. Eliminate, or deactivate, it.

3. Prevent its return by gentle passive stretching of the muscle to maintain its full normal stretch length.

4. Eliminate perpetuating factors in your body and in your life that keep the problem going. Since poor posture is a major cause of continuing pain from trigger points, we will address posture after you have studied the muscle groups.

You will see some X marks on the drawings. These are the sites of the trigger points. The clusters of dots indicate where the pain is felt, and the darkest areas indicate the major site of pain.

Splenius Cervicus (Back of Neck)

The splenius cervicus runs down from the back of the neck to in between the shoulder blades (figure 3.1). Activation of trigger points in this muscle is often due to direct trauma, such as a whiplash injury or blow to the head. Sometimes holding the head and neck in a forward, crooked position for a prolonged period can also cause triggers. Bending over a desk or computer is a common culprit. This muscle is especially vulnerable when exposed to a cold draft. Pain from this muscle is referred from the back of the neck upward through the head to the back of the eye and causes neck pain and blurred vision.

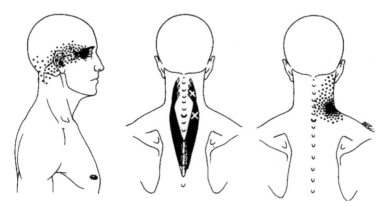

Figure 3.1. Splenius Cervicus

Sternocleidomastoid (Under the Ear)

The sternocleidomastoid, or SCM, contains two parts that attach to the mastoid bone: one part connects to the collarbone and the other to the breastbone (sternum). SCM trigger points can be caused by trauma, looking up for long periods of time, or putting too much stress on your muscles. Even the compression of a tight collar can cause trigger points, as can poorly designed work areas, such as those with a keyboard or counter that is too high. Sitting in poorly designed chairs or other furniture can also cause triggers to develop.

The sternal portion (see figure 3.2a) can refer pain to the front or top of the head, over the eye, across the cheek, or to the back of the throat and tongue. A trigger can cause pain deep inside the eye or ear, causing tearing, reddening of the eye, or drooping of the eyelid. It can also cause visual disturbances such as blurring of vision. Ringing in the ear and even deafness have also been reported.

The collarbone attachment (see figure 3.2b) can cause frontal headaches and earaches, and pain to the cheek and back teeth. Other symptoms are dizziness caused by movement and disturbed balance, dizziness from improper posture, frontal headaches and impaired sleep. Spatial disorientation and vertigo are common. Episodes of dizziness can last for seconds or hours. Loss of motor coordination can happen unexpectedly.

Starlanyl (1997) cautions, "Any chronic infection, sinusitis, dental problems, or uncorrected vision should be dealt with promptly. The neck holds the secret to most dizziness. However, dizziness can be caused by other medical problems; so check with your doctor."

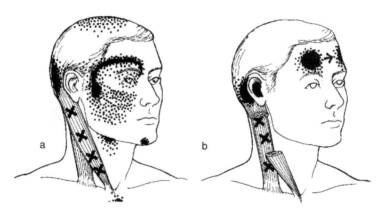

Figure 3.2. Sternocleidomastoid

Trapezius (On Top of the Shoulder)

The trapezius extends across your back and shoulders (figure 3.3). Trigger points are often activated by trauma from whiplash or other injuries, holding hands above waist level to work, weight of a heavy coat or shoulder bag, poor postural habits, or a tight bra strap. A trigger point in this muscle is a major source of tension headaches. Pain is referred to the back and side of the neck, behind the ear and up to the temple. Sometimes there can be pain in the lower back teeth and even the outer ear. If you sleep with a thick, firm pillow this muscle is especially vulnerable to trigger points.

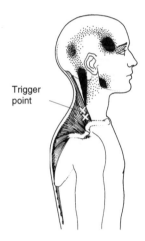
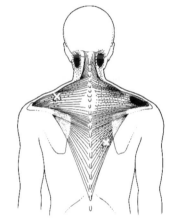

Figure 3.3. Trapezius

Masseter (Cheek Muscle)

This muscle is just below and in front of your ear. Trigger points are often activated by repeatedly grinding or clenching your teeth, sucking your thumb, chewing gum, cracking hard substances with your teeth, having a poor bite, breathing through your mouth, a nasal obstruction, or prolonged dental work. Chronic overwork and other major stresses in your life can also cause you to clench. Holding the jaw in other than a normal rest position for prolonged periods will make the pain worse. Tell your dentist to allow you to exercise your jaws intermittently during dental work.

Figure 3.4 shows the different pain patterns caused by this muscle:

- Pain is referred to the upper back teeth, adjacent gums, front of the face and under the eye (a). This maxillary (upper jaw) pain may feel like sinusitis.

- Trigger points refer pain to the lower back molars and jaw (b). Referred pain to a tooth can also cause sensitivity to heat and cold as well as pressure.

- Trigger points projecting pain in an arc that extends across the temple and over the eyebrow (c). Pain is also referred to the lower jaw.

- Trigger points in the deep layer of the masseter send pain to the cheek and temporomandibular joint, and deep into the ear causing ringing or roaring (d). This trigger point often causes a deep, maddening itch in the ear.

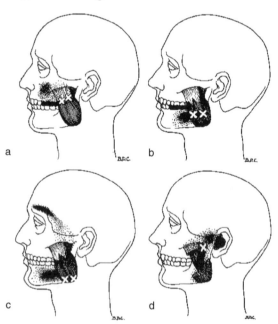

Figure 3.4. Masseter

Medial Pterygoid (Inside the Jaw)

Trigger points in this area cause difficulty in swallowing and painful, moderately-restricted jaw opening. They can also be responsible for pain in your tongue, roof of your mouth, back of your nasal cavity, floor of your nose, your throat, and deep in your ear. Stuffiness in the ear is common because this muscle helps keep your auditory tubes closed. Pain increases when you try to open your mouth wide, chew food, or clench your teeth. You feel soreness inside your throat and it hurts when you swallow. Anxiety and emotional tensions worsen these symptoms as does chronic infection in the area.

Figure 3.5a shows pain being referred to the tongue, roof of the mouth, below and behind the temporomandibular joint, deep in the ear, and on the floor of the nose and throat. Trigger points in this muscle can cause ear stuffiness, difficulty swallowing and moderately-restricted jaw opening. Figure 3.5b is an anatomical cutaway that shows the location of the internal trigger point in the muscle.

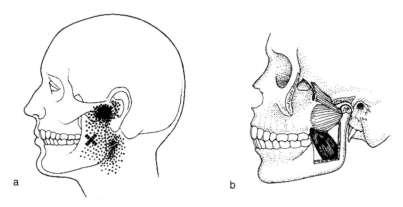

a   b

Figure 3.5. Medial Pterygoid

Lateral Pterygoid (Behind the Upper Third Molars)

This muscle is the chief source of referred pain in the temporomandibular area. Trigger points refer pain deep into the temporomandibular joint and to the maxillary sinus. The trigger points are caused by and can cause bruxism (grinding while clenching). When tense, the lateral pterygoid can be responsible for functional disorders of the jaw joint. Figure 3.6b shows an internal view of the muscle.

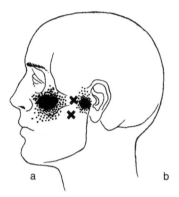
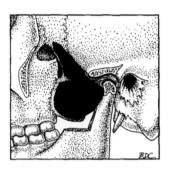

a   b

Figure 3.6. Lateral Pterygoid

Temporalis (Side of Head)

Activation of trigger points in this muscle may be due to long periods of jaw immobilization (open or closed), clenching your teeth, direct trauma, gum chewing, breathing through your mouth, or exposure to cold drafts. Temporalis trigger points refer pain over the eyebrow, to the upper teeth, throughout the temple area, and behind the eye. You may feel that your bite is off. Your teeth may also be sensitive to heat, cold, and touch.

Each temporalis trigger point has a different referral pattern. Figure 3.7 will help you understand specific referral patterns:

- Trigger points in the front portion (a) will frequently refer pain to front teeth (feels similar to a bad toothache), over the eyebrow, and behind the eye.

- Trigger points in the middle portion (b and c) refer pain to the middle and back teeth.

- Trigger points in the back portion of this muscle (d) will often refer pain to the back of the head.

Over the years I have seen many patients who did not understand where the pain in their teeth was coming from. They'd had one tooth after another removed, only to have the trigger point pain continue. This should never happen. Trigger points should always be suspected when obvious causes of toothache cannot be found.

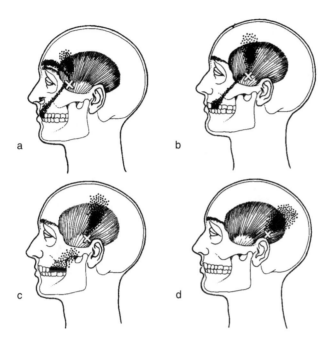

Figure 3.7. Temporalis

Levator Scapulae (Side of the Neck)

Trigger points in the levator scapulae (figure 3.8) can result from postural, psychological, or activity stress. They cause what is commonly referred to as a "stiff neck." The pain produced is concentrated along the inside border of the shoulder blade and can project to the rear of the shoulder joint. Patients are usually unable to turn their heads. Instead, they must turn their bodies to look behind.

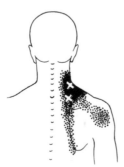

Figure 3.8. Levator Scapulae

What You Can Do about Referred Pain

By now you have probably located a few trigger points in your body that are causing pain. Now that you know what is causing this pain, you're ready to learn what you can do about it. This involves eliminating or deactivating the trigger point, preventing its return by gentle, passive stretching, and eliminating the bad habits that keep the problem going. Because there are not many health care professionals who are trained in trigger point therapy, you may have a hard time finding someone who is qualified to assist you in this process. Treatments such as physical therapy, Myotherapy, Myofascial Release, and home care remedies, however, can be helpful.

Physical Therapy

Physical therapists are key in treating TMJ disorder and probably have the greatest availability of procedures of any discipline. Physical therapy modalities are described in detail in chapter 10.

You may have heard about a therapy called Spray and Stretch: A vaporcoolant is sprayed on the affected area to prevent the muscle from tensing. Then the clinician gently stretches the muscle, a little at a time, to release the spasm. Passive stretching of the affected muscle is crucial to the success of Spray and Stretch. This technique should only be done by a properly trained clinician.

Myotherapy

You may want to find a person who is trained in a procedure called Myotherapy. This technique was developed by a physical therapist named Bonnie Prudden. In 1977, she wrote a national bestseller called *Pain Erasure: The Bonnie Prudden Way*. In this book she provides diagrams of the pain patterns in the various muscles and gives instructions on how to deactivate the triggers. She also suggests exercises to prevent the return of the triggers. I call it a recipe book on trigger points and recommend the book to all of my patients with TMJ disorder. If you are unable to find a certified Bonnie Prudden Myotherapist, Prudden's book will help you "do it yourself" at home. You may wish to contact her "Help Line": Bonnie Prudden Pain Erasure Clinic, 7800 E. Speedway, Tucson, AZ 85710, (520) 529-3979.

Myofascial Release

Another helpful therapy that I strongly recommend is called Myofascial Release (MFR). This therapy, which was discussed briefly in chapter 1, was developed by John Barnes, a physical therapist. Barnes has two training centers and teaches this technique to physicians, dentists, chiropractors, physical therapists, and other interested people. It is a gentle technique and can be effective with people who have severe pain. Many people with TMJ disorder, especially fibromyalgia patients, cannot tolerate anything beyond this very gentle, featherlike touch. This therapy provides both physical release of the spasms and an accompanying emotional release.

You can check with your local physical therapy centers and chiropractors to see if anyone in your area is trained in this technique.

Home Care Remedies

Using the information in this chapter, you can find your trigger points yourself. In order to deactivate them, press or rub them for seven to ten seconds, or until you feel the spasm release. You may need a friend to help you get to some hard-to-reach areas. However, the most important part of doing it yourself is the gentle, passive stretch that is required to bring the muscle back from its shortened state to its normal resting length. Failure to do this will simply cause the muscle to go back into spasm. Applying moist heat to the area of the trigger point for twenty minutes after such an exercise can be helpful and feels good.

The most important home remedy is correcting bad habits and faulty posture, which I address in the next chapter. So, read on and pay close attention.

4

Eliminate Harmful Habits

If you want to take charge of your healing, eliminating harmful habits is one of the most important tasks you can perform. Harmful habits, which serve as perpetuating factors, not only contribute to your TMJ disorder, but they also prevent you from getting and staying well. No one else in your life is aware of what you are doing to perpetuate your problem, so you are the only one who can control this part of your wellness plan. Think about it this way: A dentist can diagnose your problem, provide a splint if necessary, adjust your occlusion if that is needed, or medicate you. A physician can prescribe medications and screen you for other physical problems. A physical therapist can give you treatments and exercises that will help alleviate your pain. A dietitian can work out the perfect nutrition program for you. But only you can assure that these interventions will be successful. Nobody can do it for you.

Bill, a sixty-year-old business owner, sought emergency help for clicking, pain in front of his right ear, and severe pain in his sinuses. He had already had sinus surgery, which he described as a "horrible experience that provided no help." Since another sinus surgery had been recommended, Bill was desperate to find a nonsurgical treatment for his problem.

My examination of Bill revealed a myofascial trigger point in the lateral pterygoid muscle (see figure 3.6). This muscle, when in spasm, is the chief cause of pain referred to the temporomandibular joint and also to the maxillary sinuses (these are the sinuses that attach to the upper jaw bone). In addition to going through the traditional dental procedures to treat TMJ disorder, Bill and I talked about certain harmful habits that were preventing him from getting well. His poor posture and gum chewing, for example, were preventing him from eliminating his trigger point. Once he understood how these habits were perpetuating his problem, he worked hard to break them. In fact, Bill was one of my star pupils in my early years of working with TMJ. He and I learned together. I followed Bill's progress for thirteen years, and he continued to be symptom-free for both TMJ disorder and sinus problems. His hard work paid off.

Harmful habits can be broken down into a few general categories: oral, postural, muscular, and nutritional. Your list of harmful habits from chapter 1 will be helpful to you as you work through this step. You may even find other contributing factors to add to your list.

Oral Habits

Oral habits include all of the things you do in and around the jaw, head, and neck area. According to Kate Hathaway, Ph.D., harmful oral habits "put strain on the temporomandibular joint and surrounding muscles that can contribute to TMJ problems and head, neck, and face pain." She suggests the following as some common harmful oral habits:

- Clenching of the teeth—day or night

- Nighttime grinding of the teeth

- Gum chewing

- Chewing on one side of the mouth only

- Incorrect posture of the tongue

- Incorrect head and neck posture

- Holding objects in the teeth, such as pencils, pens, paper clips, etc.

- Pencil chewing

- Nail biting

- Cradling of the phone between the neck and shoulder

- Biting the insides of the cheek

Hathaway found that

> These habits, when they occur often over a long period of time put continual strain on the joints and muscles of the head, neck, and jaw. When a person clenches, for example, the jaw and neck muscles contract (tighten) and this increases the force on the jaw joints. Even when the teeth don't touch, a jaw tightening habit can put considerable force against the muscles and joints.
>
> If these habits only occurred once, this might not be a problem—but then they wouldn't be habits either! It is the continual "microtraumas" to the joints and muscles that eventually will take their toll on the structures of the face, head, and neck, and can even change jaw, head, and neck posture more (which then continues to "microtraumatize" the structure). While a "macrotrauma," like an injury, can also result in TMJ problems and muscle pain, the "microtraumatic" habits like those listed will put too much long-term strain on the joints and muscles and can result in the same kind of pain.
>
> Four out of five TMJ "problems" involve only muscle problems rather than joint problems and can be effectively managed by working with the muscles and by discontinuing the habits that continually put strain on the system. Whatever the problem (joint or muscle, or both), it is vital to work with the muscles and habits that traumatize the structures. When the health of the joints in the body are continually threatened by such "microtraumas" or "macrotraumas," the muscles and ligaments around the joint will automatically tighten to protect the joint. In turn, however, the muscles will begin to be traumatized and will also hurt and begin to function abnormally. It is for a similar reason that we injure any other body joint (e.g., a knee or ankle). We subject the joint to incorrect forces which, if prolonged, will traumatize and potentially injure that joint. This, then, may lead to a sprain of ligaments, a muscle sprain, or a combination, as the muscles and ligaments are forced to work in ways that they aren't designed to (e.g., when an ankle is twisted).

Nighttime Habits

Because you do not learn new behaviors in your sleep, it is more than likely that if you clench your jaw or grind your teeth while you sleep at night, you also do it during the day. Since at night you are literally unconscious, recognizing these habits and trying to break them won't be very effective. You must instead try to break these habits during the day. Once you do that, you'll find the nighttime habits will also be affected.

Postural Habits

In *The Atlas of Temporomandibular Orthopedics*, Steven Smith (1981) reported on the relationship that was found to exist between jaw dysfunction and poor posture. Although it is often overlooked, total body posture is a major factor in TMJ disorder. When you're dealing with TMJ disorder, you'd expect to be primarily concerned with your head and neck muscles. However, since trigger points are present throughout the body, how you stand, sit, walk, sleep, play, and work can make a world of difference in how your jaw feels. Poor posture can actually cause fascia to malfunction (as can illness, surgery, or inflammation). When this happens, the fascia becomes tight and binds down, resulting in abnormal pressure on nerves, muscles, bones, or organs of the body. Since fascia is interconnected throughout the entire body, a problem in one area can affect more than just that area. That is why I have all patients mark on a diagram where they have pain—from head to toe. You did this in chapter 1.

You might be wondering, "What business does a dentist have meddling with a person's posture? Shouldn't a dentist stick to the teeth and jaws, since that's where his training was focused?" Herein lies the problem. When we professionals fail to look at the total patient, head to toe, and to consider all of the factors contributing to the jaw problem, our treatments fail, and the patient does not get well.

There are various theories on the relationship of body posture to jaw imbalance, TMJ disorders, and craniofacial pain. Some authorities feel that jaw imbalance causes postural changes in the total body. Others feel that postural imbalances contribute to the pain and disability of TMJ disorder. You are caught in the middle somewhere. I highly respect these professionals; but I think that from your perspective, it really doesn't matter all that much which comes first. What does matter is that you understand that proper body alignment affects the healthy functioning of your entire body.

Many years ago, I had a number of patients who failed to respond regardless of what treatments I prescribed. This was before I understood the importance of the connection between total posture and the jaw joints. Once I incorporated that concept into my treatment plan, patient success soared.

Robin McKenzie, a physiotherapist from Wellington, New Zealand, is an international authority on back and neck problems. With his permission, I am summarizing parts of, and adapting drawings from, his two outstanding books—*Treat Your Own Neck* and *Treat Your Own Back*—to give you a brief, simple visual understanding of some common harmful postural habits and how you should correct them. (See appendix A for information on obtaining these books.)

Standing Posture

Standing properly might seem like something that should just come naturally, but if the position in figure 4.1b looks a little too familiar to you, then your standing posture might need some adjustment. Proper standing posture (see figure 4.1a) involves an inward curve in the small of your back. This hollow in the lower back is called *lumbar lordosis,* or *lumbar curve*; it follows the natural contour of the spine. The same is true of the inward curve at the base of your neck, just above the shoulder girdle. This curve is called *cervical lordosis,* or *cervical curve*. The goal for proper posture is to maintain the inward curves in these areas as much as possible when standing and, in fact, in all of your activities. Sometimes your job or a recreational activity makes this task virtually impossible, especially if you need to stand for a long period of time. When lordosis is lost, through slouching or bending for long periods of time, back pain can result. If corrections are not made, permanent damage can occur.

The "Mountain Pose," a starting exercise in Yoga that is described in chapter 6, will help you attain better posture and balance.

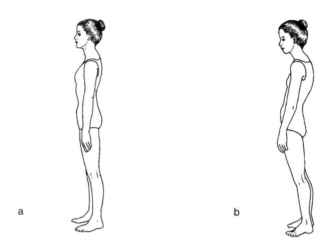

Figure 4.1. Standing Posture

Walking

Walking is a wonderful way to relax and exercise, but not if your head is protruded and your shoulders are slumped over as in figure 4.2. Next time you're at the mall, observe how people walk. Is it any wonder back pain is such a universal problem? Remember, the head weighs nine to fifteen pounds, and if it is not positioned correctly on top of the spine, the whole body becomes unbalanced. The man in figure 4.2 needs to learn to straighten up, bring his shoulders up and back, and use the strength of his neck to hold his head up.

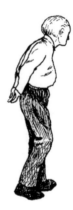

Figure 4.2. Bad Walking Posture

Lifting

There are countless times when you find yourself bending over to pick something up. Some people have jobs that require lifting heavy objects. Others need to lift boxes, laundry baskets, or other objects from the house. The woman in figure 4.3 is sure to hurt herself lifting the box that way. Always try to remember to keep some lordosis in your lower back, bend from your knees rather than your waist, hold the object as close to your body as possible, lean back, and stay in balance as you lift the load. If you need to turn, shift your feet to avoid twisting your lower back.

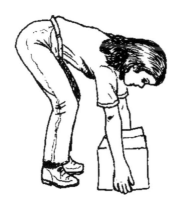

Figure 4.3. Bad Lifting Posture

Working in Stooped Positions

Vacuuming, raking, bed making, and gardening are a few of the tasks you do at home in a stooped position. These activities frequently cause you to bend and twist improperly, thus placing undue pressure on the lower back. Many occupations require this type of posture as well.

According to McKenzie, if you must be in a stooped position, try to take breaks from the posture regularly. You can do this simply by standing up and doing the Back Stretch described at the end of this section (and depicted in figure 4.16) every few minutes. Doing this stretch even before you begin to stoop can be helpful, too.

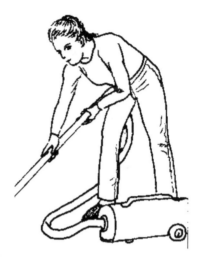

Figure 4.4. Stooped Position

Sitting Posture

When walking briskly, you usually assume a fairly upright posture. The head is retracted and held directly over the vertebral column and it consequently receives the maximum support possible. When you sit and relax in a chair, however, frequently the head and neck slowly protrude because the muscles that support them become tired. As the muscles tire they relax and you lose the main support for good posture. The result is protruded head posture (as in figures 4.5b and 4.14). This posture is very common. It is not present during infancy, but develops from the mid-teens on. This may have to do with the fact that your body is not really designed to be seated for six to eight hours daily.

The goal for proper sitting posture is to maintain the inward curve in the lower back (lordosis) when you sit (as in figure 4.5a), and to periodically interrupt the position by standing or walking around briefly. Sitting properly is more easily accomplished if you have some support in the small of your back, such as a lumbar roll as shown in figure 4.5a.

Here are some more common harmful sitting habits:

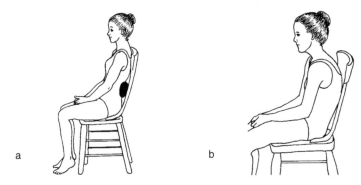

Figure 4.5. Sitting Posture

Rounded Back

People with sedentary office jobs easily develop low back problems, as they often sit with a rounded back for hours on end. Prolonged poor sitting posture (as in figure 4.6b) will cause an overstretching of the ligaments. Any job or activity that requires you to hold your head or body in a static or slumped position for long periods of time puts you at risk for back and neck problems. When working at your desk, make sure your lower back is supported so the natural curve is maintained, your feet are flat on the floor, the height of your desk is such that your shoulders can be relaxed, and your forearms are level or tilted slightly upward. Get up and move around briefly every half hour. Assembly line workers or precision workers who do constant, repetitious work (as in figure 4.7) also need to try to get up and move around at regular intervals during the workday. McKenzie's Back Stretch exercise that is included at the end of this section (figure 4.16) is very helpful to people in these situations.

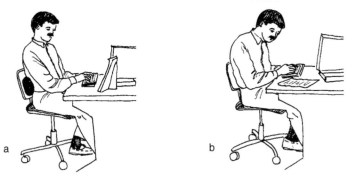

Figure 4.6. Working at a Desk

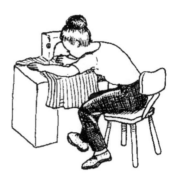

Figure 4.7. Slumping over Your Work

Phone Position

Do you see yourself in figure 4.8? With the advent of portable phones we can do any number of jobs with the phone propped on our shoulders. This can actually be done sitting or standing. Keeping the head bent for an extended period of time can put a great strain on the muscles and ligaments in the neck, causing pain and discomfort. You might find yourself in this position at work or at home. Try to avoid it as much as possible.

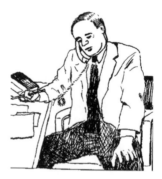

Figure 4.8. Neck Holding Phone

Asleep in the Chair

Do you ever fall asleep in your chair or on your couch at night with your head or back in an awkward position as in figure 4.9? If this happens frequently, it will become a major cause of back and neck pain problems that won't go away. Note the depth of the seat of your favorite chair or couch. If it is too long, your back will naturally slump. If you are not able to replace the furniture, you will need to use firm cushions or a lumbar roll to get your back in the right position to provide the proper lumbar support.

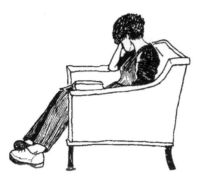

Figure 4.9. Asleep in the Chair

On the Couch

I would guess that nine out of every ten people look like the man in figure 4.10 when they come home from work and sit down to read the paper or watch TV. How about you? This is a habit not easily broken. However, if you can develop the technique of supporting your lower back with cushions or a lumbar roll, you will soon feel so much better that you will search out the proper support each time you sit.

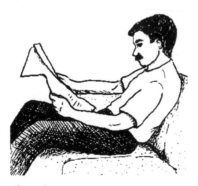

Figure 4.10. On the Couch

Reading in Bed

Am I taking all of the fun out of your life by suggesting that reading in bed in the position shown in figure 4.11 is bad for you? (Note the crooked neck and rounded back.) Unfortunately, most people love to relax in this position and do it frequently. But this posture only perpetuates the problem, from a bad back or painful neck to TMJ pain. You can alleviate this problem by using firm support under your back and neck to achieve a straight line from head to hips. Providing support under the knees, as shown, is important also.

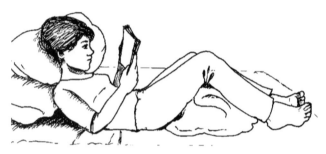

Figure 4.11. Reading in Bed

Driving

Think for a minute how you sit when you're in a car. Does the posture in figure 4.12 look familiar to you? See how her head is protruded and back is flat? Many car makers today are becoming more concerned about the design of their seats. In fact, the McKenzie Institute was asked by Toyota to provide expertise in the design of new seating for a number of their vehicles.

If you experience back pain because of your car seat, a lumbar roll or small, rolled-up towel could help keep your back in the proper position. Always remember to keep your head properly positioned and balanced on top of the spine, and keep a moderate lordosis in the lumbar area. On a long trip, be sure to stop frequently to stretch and walk around a bit.

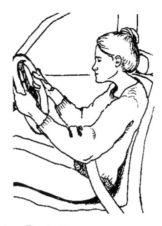

Figure 4.12. Bad Driving Posture

Sitting without Back Support

How many moms and dads have spent hours in the bleachers watching a child's game? Or, if you engage in sports, you might find yourself sitting out an inning on the bench. Sitting with the back unsupported as in figure 4.13 for long periods of time can result in back, neck, and TMJ pain.

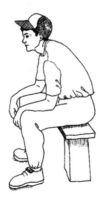

Figure 4.13. Sitting without Back Support

Relaxing after Vigorous Activity

Many people complain of back pain after engaging in some vigorous activity, such as running, biking, playing football or tennis. It is easy to attribute such pains to these activities. But usually what happens is that we sit and relax after such activity, often collapsing slouched in a chair. McKenzie finds that thoroughly exercised joints of the spine distort easily if they are placed in a slouched position for long periods. Always stretch for a few minutes after you exercise in order to avoid this pitfall. Also, after vigorous activity you should retract and extend the head and neck five or six times. In other words, push your head forward and then pull your head back five or six times. When you sit down to rest, you should avoid the protruded head posture (as in figure 4.14).

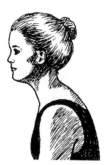

Figure 4.14. Protruded Head Posture

Sleeping Posture

Some people like to sleep on their stomachs and frequently wake up with pain in the neck or headache, which wears off as the day progresses. In this position, the head is usually turned to one side (as in figure 4.15), and some of the joints, especially in the upper neck, reach the maximum possible degree of turning, or may come close to it. Consequently, this position places great strain on the soft tissues surrounding the joints of the neck and those between the upper neck and the head. If you have problems of this nature, you must avoid lying face down. Sleeping on your back may be hard to get used to at first, but it'll help ease some of your jaw and neck pain.

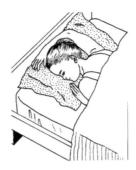

Figure 4.15. Bad Sleeping Posture

The Back Stretch

When you find yourself sitting or standing improperly, or for a prolonged period, this stretch will help you relieve the pressure on your lower back and help to restore the lost lordosis. Place your hands in the small of your back with fingers pointing backward. Keep your knees straight and bend backward as far as is comfortable. Hold the position for a second or two and then return to the starting position. As you continue to do this exercise, you will be able to finally extend to the full position, as shown in figure 4.16. Repeat two or three times if it feels comfortable.

As a preventive measure, repeat the exercise every once in a while whenever you find yourself working in a forward bent position. McKenzie suggests also doing this exercise before prolonged sitting or standing.

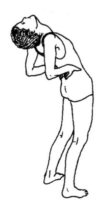

Figure 4.16. The Back Exercise

When pains of postural origin are first felt, merely correcting your posture easily eliminates them. As time passes, however, if uncorrected, the habitual poor posture causes changes to the structure and shape of the joints, excessive wear occurs, and premature aging of the joints is a consequence. The effect of poor posture in the long term, therefore, can be just as severe and harmful as the effects of injury. Those who allow poor posture to persist throughout their lifetime become bent and stooped as they age. When called upon to straighten and stand erect, they are unable to comply. When asked to turn their heads, they are unable to do so.

Deformities in the elderly are the visible effect of poor postural habits. There are secondary and sometimes severe consequences when these habits affect their organs: the lungs are constricted, and breathing is affected as the back becomes bent; the stomach and other internal organs are deprived of their correct support and may well be affected adversely.

McKenzie feels that the bent, stooped posture considered by many to be one of the inevitable consequences of aging is not at all inevitable and the time to commence preventive action is now. One action you could take is doing the Back Stretch exercise at least once a day.

Abuse of Muscles and Nutritional Habits

Muscle abuse can be caused by lack of exercise just as it can be caused by too strenuous exercise. Muscles atrophy when not used. That's why people who are confined to wheelchairs or beds are greatly helped when provided with adaptive exercises. On the other hand, the old adage "no pain, no gain" in your exercise program is equally harmful to your muscles. Sustained vigorous exercise may be good for your heart, but be aware of what your body is telling you when your muscles tire and exhaustion sets in.

Your body also sends you messages about your nutritional habits. It's true, you are what you eat. But each person's body has different nutritional needs, and accepts or rejects nutrients differently. Calcium, iron, and potassium deficiencies are often found in TMJ disorder patients. Special attention should be given to your overall nutritional program as well as focusing on these particular nutrients.

Chapter 6 has all the information you need about exercise and nutrition. When you read that information, however, keep in mind the suggestions in this chapter for eliminating harmful habits.

Breaking the Habit

Your bad habits will not go away by themselves. The first step in eliminating harmful habits is to understand that *you* are in control, not the habit. Once you can accept that, you're ready for the rest of the process, which involves

1. Becoming more aware of the habit

2. Knowing why it's necessary to correct the habit

3. Knowing how to correct the habit (for instance, what to do with the teeth and tongue, how to hold your head and neck)

4. Making a commitment to monitor the bad habit and replace it with a healthy habit until the healthy one becomes second nature

The beginning of this chapter has helped you with the first three parts of the process. The last step, however, is by far the most important one for you to do on your own. While your health care professional can help you become more aware of your habit and what to do about it, he or she can't follow you every day to make sure you're actually putting your habit-breaking knowledge to use. Nobody can make you change if you don't want to. And change won't take place unless you work to make it happen.

Now that you've read about some harmful habits, are you ready to design your own strategy for eliminating yours? You filled out a checklist similar to the following one when you identified some perpetuating factors in the questionnaire in chapter 1. Turn back to that list and review the perpetuating factors that you indicated pertain to you. Did you miss any? In the following list of harmful habits, check off those that you've already indicated as well as any that you may have missed the first time around.

Oral habits

_____ Gum chewing

_____ Cheek chewing

_____ Clenching

_____ Bruxing (grinding teeth)

_____ Pencil biting

_____ Nail biting

_____ Incorrect posture of tongue

_____ Chewing on objects

_____ Holding objects between the teeth (such as pencils, pens, etc.)

_____ Chewing on one side only

_____ Pushing the tongue against teeth

_____ Sucking on candy

_____ Tightening of facial muscles (such as frowning or grimacing)

_____ Other: _____

Postural habits

_____ Leaning over a desk

_____ Holding the phone on your shoulder

_____ Poor posture while working at the computer

_____ Lifting improperly

_____ Slouching on the couch

_____ Sleeping on stomach

_____ Reading in bed with neck bent

_____ Sleeping on a bulky or bouncy pillow

_____ Improper bending

_____ Head protruded

_____ Slouching while walking

_____ Poor posture while driving

_____ Crossing one leg over another while sitting

____ Sitting in ill-fitting furniture

____ Prolonged immobility

____ Other: _____

Abuse of muscles and bad nutritional habits (See chapter 6)

____ Overstressing muscles in exercise

____ Constricting pressure on muscles

____ Low levels of B_1, B_6, B_{12}, and folic acid

____ Vitamin C deficiency

____ Calcium, potassium, and iron deficiencies

____ Poor diet in general

____ Too much caffeine

____ Other: _____

Now that you've identified them, it's time to prioritize your harmful habits. Start by listing in any order the items that you checked off. Leave the shorter line on the left of each line blank for now.

These are my particular habits that I need to work on:

____ _____

____ _____

____ _____

____ _____

____ _____

____ _____

____ _____

____ _____

____ _____

Number your list from easiest to most difficult using the blank lines to the left of each habit. You'll put a 1 next to the habit you think will be the easiest to change, a 2 next to the second easiest, and so on all the way to the most difficult to change. By now, you suspect my devious plot, don't you? It simply makes sense to achieve some success quickly; so tackle the habits that are easiest to change first, and then work your way down the list. You can set goals for yourself using the following four-column list. For example, if gum chewing is one of your habits, you may fill the list in like this:

Harmful Habit   **Timeline for Change**

	1 month	*3 months*	*6 months*
Chewing gum	Cut down to 2 packs of gum a week	Only chew gum when commuting to work	Only chew gum as an occasional treat

Now it's your turn.

Harmful Habit   **Timeline for Change**

	1 month	*3 months*	*6 months*
_____	_____	_____	_____
_____	_____	_____	_____
_____	_____	_____	_____
_____	_____	_____	_____
_____	_____	_____	_____
_____	_____	_____	_____
_____	_____	_____	_____
_____	_____	_____	_____
_____	_____	_____	_____

Once you've set your goals, make sure you understand why you need to break certain habits and how, physically, to correct those habits. Then, you must devise your own ways to break these harmful habits. It probably won't be easy; but it may not be as hard as you think. Awareness itself is a big part of facilitating change.

A simple yet effective technique Dr. Hathaway uses for breaking harmful oral habits (it can work with other habits as well, especially posture), is to monitor your oral habits every twenty minutes. A simple kitchen timer can be used to keep track of the time. She says,

> If [you find your] teeth together, the jaw malpositioned, or [note] poor head, neck, or tongue posture, [you should] immediately correct the error (tongue up, teeth apart, muscles relaxed) and continue with the daily routine until the next monitoring period. In some cases, the problem may not involve tooth contact, but may involve an "unconscious" habit of tightening the facial muscles such as frowning, grimacing, biting the insides of the cheek or tongue. This regular monitoring and correcting results in a positive alternative to the clenching and other habits, and the habit reverses itself by the consistent retraining approach. In essence, [you learn] an alternative, improved behavior that is incompatible with clenching. When the monitoring and correcting approach has been consistent, a habit can be effectively changed in a short time, and with continued monitoring will be maintained for a long period. This approach is simple and straightforward but requires [your] commitment to change behaviors and to assume self-responsibility. It is surprisingly effective for the majority of patients with oral habits, and the results last as long as the individual remains conscientious about maintaining correct tongue and teeth position. If the habit reappears, the same monitoring approach should be used again.
>
> Other behaviors that contribute to muscle tightening include poor posture, grimacing, gum chewing, unilateral chewing, candy sucking, nail biting, and object chewing. It is important to [be educated] about what specifically needs to be changed and why. It is not enough [if your doctor tells you,] "You have to stop chewing gum." [You need] to understand that gum chewing requires muscle force that is excessive for the jaw structures, and has a significant negative impact on muscle contraction and the temporomandibular joint. When [a] patient understands the consequences of the habit, willingness to comply with treatment increases dramatically.

Here are a few things to keep in mind when you're trying to break bad habits:

- Tackle the bad habits one at a time.

- Start with the easiest and work your way down your list.

- Don't become discouraged if you don't succeed right away. Take it one day at a time.

If you become discouraged, you will be tempted to quit and revert back to your old ways. That would be a real shame considering what you are going through. You are in pain now or else you wouldn't be reading this book. You have the opportunity to help yourself. Let that be your main goal.

Remember that the professionals working with you can help identify problem areas and do what they do best for you; but you will be the final judge of your success. You are the only one who can see the total picture. After all, confidence in your treatment plan is powerful medicine. You can do it. I know you can.

5

Identify Stressors

Although experts still disagree on what exactly causes TMJ disorder, most agree that stress is, at the very least, a contributing factor. People with TMJ disorder often clench or grind their teeth, which can tire the jaw muscles and lead to pain. There is no consensus, however, on whether stress is the cause of the clenching/grinding and subsequent jaw pain, or the result of dealing with chronic pain or dysfunction. It's possible that both are true, and stress and TMJ disorder feed off of each other in a vicious cycle. So while stress does not actually cause TMJ disorder, it can exacerbate some of the symptoms. In turn, the pain and discomfort of the disorder surely contributes to your stress level. It's important to remember that stress is a factor in everyday life and is not bad in and of itself. It is how you react to the stress that matters. Your understanding of how you cope with stress will help in the healing process.

Sandra, an eighteen-year-old single mother of an infant child, came into the office complaining of sharp, excruciating, constant pain inside her right ear. In addition, she experienced headaches, dizziness, back and neck pain, and ringing in her right ear. She said she often started the day out with a headache—before she even got out of bed. As we went over her symptoms, Sandra reported fatigue, soreness in and around her jaw, numbness in her fingers, difficulty sleeping, and pressure behind the eyes. She said she'd been feeling "stressed out and depressed" lately and had been biting her nails more often, chewing more gum, and had noticed a new tendency to bite the inside of her cheek. She had also lost some weight because of a decrease in appetite.

Sandra had supportive family members. In fact, they sent her to seven specialists within a month in their desperate search to find a solution to her many problems. She saw an orthodontist, who removed her orthodontic bands; two ear, nose, and throat specialists; an oral surgeon, who suspected TMJ disorder; a psychiatrist, who recognized her stress level and hospitalized her for eighteen days; a general dentist, who made a retainer; and a physical therapist, who recognized TMJ disorder, and referred Sandra to me. Each specialist concentrated on his or her own particular area of expertise; but none saw the total picture.

Sandra was pleased that someone could finally diagnose her problem and was eager to participate in her treatment plan. In addition to discussing her symptoms and harmful habits, we talked about how the stress in her life was contributing to her problem. Understanding her reactions to stressful situations was an important part of this process. Soon enough, she understood her total problem, head to toe. She faithfully began doing her exercises and learning about stress reduction strategies. Sandra was free of symptoms within six months and continues to be fine two years later.

An unusual case? Not at all! All patients report multiple symptoms. That's why diagnosis is so difficult and why patients frequently move from specialist to specialist in search of relief. With all of the different symptoms people with TMJ disorder report, is it any wonder that professionals have difficulty diagnosing this elusive problem? In Sandra's case, except for the symptoms around the jaw, the other symptoms could have been caused by any number of diseases.

What Is Stress?

Simply defined, *stress* is any factor in your environment—good or bad—that you must adjust to. When the demands in your life are greater than your ability to meet those demands, you start to feel stressed. Such demands are called *stressors*: they are those events and conditions in your life that cause stress. Stressors vary from person to person. What is stressful to one person may be routine or even enjoyable to another. Some are minor irritations in daily living that grate on the nerves. Other stressors are serious life events over which we may have no control. Death of a spouse or close family member, marital problems, loss of a job or frustration at work, financial problems, personal injury or illness, and illness of a family member are a few examples.

Researchers generally agree that the following events in a person's life result in the greatest stress levels. They are listed in order of intensity (Gelb 1980, 3).

1. Death of a spouse

2. Divorce

3. Marital separation

4. Detention in jail or other institution

5. Death of a close family member

6. Major personal injury or illness

7. Marriage

8. Getting fired from a job

9. Marital reconciliation

10. Retirement from work

11. Major change in health or behavior of a family member

12. Pregnancy

13. Sexual difficulties

14. Gaining a new family member (through birth, adoption, a family member moving in, etc.)

15. Major business readjustment

16. Major change in financial state (e.g., a lot worse off or a lot better off than usual)

17. Death of a close friend

18. Changing to a different line of work

19. Major change in the number of arguments with spouse (e.g., either a lot more or a lot less than usual regarding child-rearing, personal habits, etc.)

20. Taking on a mortgage greater than $10,000 (e.g., purchasing a home, a business, etc.)

How Does the Body React to Stress?

Stress affects you not only psychologically, but also physiologically. The *stress-response mechanism*, also known as the *fight-or-flight response*, is the physical response your body has when a stressful event occurs. Once you're familiar with this concept, you will understand what actions you must take to cope with stress and avoid further damage to your body.

The human body has a built-in alarm system that is activated when a threat is present. The body's reaction is similar to that of extreme fright: the heart beats faster, blood pressure rises, and breathing becomes shallow and faster. Certain chemicals and hormones are released in the body. The body is preparing to either attack the threat (fight) or to back off (flight).

If the body is unable to adapt to the challenge of a stressor by controlling the stress response and returning to normal functioning, a state of exhaustion will occur.

How Does Prolonged Stress Affect Your Health?

New evidence is coming out every day on the adverse effects of prolonged stress on health. Here are a few of the problems it can cause:

- *Weakening of the immune system.* Cortisol produced during the stress response may suppress your immune system, increasing your susceptibility to infectious diseases. Studies suggest bacterial infections such as tuberculosis and group A streptococcal disease increase during stress. Stress may also make you prone to upper respiratory viral infections such as cold or flu.

- *Cardiovascular disease.* Under acute stress, your heart beats quickly. You're more susceptible to angina (a type of chest pain) and heart rhythm irregularities. If you are a person whose blood pressure is normal in the doctor's office, but shoots up under real-life conditions, acute stress may add to your risk of a heart attack. When stress persists, increased blood clotting as a result of the stress response can put you at risk for a heart attack or stroke.

- *Asthma.* If you have asthma, a stressful situation can bring on an attack.

- *Gastrointestinal problems.* Stress can make your symptoms worse if you have an ulcer or irritable bowel syndrome.

According to Baltzell,

- 30 to 40 percent of all medical office visits are stress related.

- Stress-related diseases cost businesses $150 billion every year.

- Stress causes high blood pressure, heart attacks, depression, addiction, tension headaches, arthritis, skin eruptions, respiratory illnesses, ulcers, irritable bowel, and PMS.

- 100 million people a week take medications for stress-related symptoms and/or diseases.

- Nearly two-thirds of companies with 750 or more employees now have stress-control programs in effect.

- Relaxed people take care of their health, get sick less often, and accomplish more.

- Even minimal time out for stress reduction each day will get results.

What Can You Do about Stress?

Every human being experiences stress. Your stress response actually protects you in some situations. You would not survive without it, so getting rid of it completely is neither possible nor desirable. Instead, you must learn some stress-coping strategies.

The amount of stress you have in your life and the way you deal with it is a very personal thing. Your physical health, emotional well-being, and available support systems at the time of a stressful event all play a part in how well you are able to cope with the stress.

Coping Strategies

You can take conscious steps to reduce some forms of stress to a manageable level and also to control your stress response. While some of the strategies might appeal to you more than others, read them all and give each a try. The strategies are

1. Set priorities

2. Assess your stressors

3. Organize your time

4. Listen to your body

5. Learn deep breathing

6. Get enough sleep

Strategy 1: Set Priorities

We all have more things to do than time in which to do them. Making a priority list can help manage these tasks. In the following three-column chart, list the tasks you need to do in the next week, placing them in the appropriate section—Essential, Important, or Optional:

Tasks That Need to Be Done

Essential	**Important**	**Optional**
Examples:	Examples:	Examples:
Go to work	*Clean house*	*Go clothes shopping*
Buy groceries	*Take car for tune-up*	*See friends*
Your list:	Your list:	Your list:
_____	_____	_____
_____	_____	_____
_____	_____	_____
_____	_____	_____
_____	_____	_____
_____	_____	_____

_____ _____ _____

_____ _____ _____

When you're planning your time, use this tasks list and keep the following in mind:

- *Essential* tasks *must* be done. Set a realistic schedule.

- *Important* tasks need to be programmed in and around essential tasks.

- Perform *optional* tasks only if and when time permits.

Setting priorities reminds me of something I learned a number of years ago from Dr. Ken Olson, author of several excellent books on stress. Ken was working with a group of dentists, and he asked us, "Does anyone ever say to you, 'You really *should* do this' or 'You *should* do that,' and it makes you feel guilty and uncomfortable because you're already doing more than you can handle?" Most of us nodded in recognition. He continued, "When this happens to you, simply respond by saying, 'Please stop *shoulding* on me!'" There was great laughter in the room that day. But believe me, this is a very effective technique that has worked well for me over the years. If you find you can't say the words out loud, say them to yourself. You will get great comfort and satisfaction as you gain control over your own life by setting your own priorities. Try not to let someone else set your priorities. Remember, also, not to *should* on yourself. Sometimes the one you're the hardest on is yourself.

Strategy 2: Assess Your Stressors

Make a list of your stressors (all of the things that really bug you or cause tension in your life). Put everything down that comes to mind, no matter how trivial it seems. (Examples: *My next door neighbor, my boss, my boyfriend/husband, my operation.*) Add to the list as things come to mind.

My Stressors

_____   _____

_____   _____

_____   _____

_____   _____

_____   _____

_____   _____

_____   _____

_____   _____

_____   _____

_____   _____

Now take the items on your list and place them into one of the following categories: Things I Can Change or Things I Can't Change.

My Personal Assessment

Things I Can Change

Examples: *Loss of job*

Marital problems

Things I Can't Change

Examples: *Death of a spouse*

Illness

Disability

_____   _____

_____   _____

_____   _____

_____   _____

_____   _____

_____   _____

_____   _____

As you look at the things you cannot change, you may realize that acceptance of the event or experience as final or irreversible can allow you to put it behind you and move on in a new direction. Don't waste a lot of time on things you cannot change. Instead, work on things you *can* change.

Strategy 3: Organize Your Time

Some people are able to do a number of things in one day, and it doesn't seem to bother them. They seem to have boundless energy and can handle a strenuous regimen quite easily. For others, this is a daunting task with stressful situations presenting themselves at every turn. Regardless of where you fall on the spectrum, you can lighten your load if you put some effort into organizing your time. Use the following suggestions:

- Do the essential tasks when you are at your peak energy level, if at all possible.

- Pace yourself and allow time for emergencies.

- Make a list of things to do so you won't forget to do something important.

- If you develop a list each day, and break it into two columns—one for things that must be done, and the other for things you would like to get done—you will have some flexibility in your day.

- Identify time wasters in your life. Think about what you do each day and work on eliminating any nonproductive activities that may be draining your energy and taking you away from the important tasks in your life.

Strategy 4: Listen to Your Body

If you listen to your body, it will let you know when you are pushing too much. If you're feeling tense, pay attention to your physical sensations. Does your neck hurt? Are your jaw muscles feeling tight? Once you've located where the tension in your body is, you can go about trying to ease it. A book like *The Daily Relaxer*, by Matthew McKay and Patrick Fanning, can help out by providing lots of relaxation strategies. Look in appendix A for information about this book.

When you feel pressured or stressed out, be good to yourself and take a little time off. Do something you really enjoy. It could be as simple as taking a walk, watching a sunset, reading a book or having lunch with a friend. But it should be something special, just for you. You will gain renewed energy from such a diversion.

Strategy 5: Learn Deep Breathing

Learning the technique of deep breathing, or relaxation breathing as it is sometimes called, is an essential tool for reducing stress. Have you ever driven on the highway and had a car suddenly pull in front of you forcing you to jam on the brakes? If you have, you understand very well what the stress-response mechanism is all about. The instant your stress-response mechanism kicks in (rapid heart beat, rise in blood pressure, and shallow, faster breathing in response to a stressful situation), you need to employ deep breathing. Once you learn to do this, you will be able to reduce your stress level no matter where you are or what you are doing.

According to Starlanyl and Copeland (1996), "Deep breathing will help to rid your body of waste gases. [It] also massages some of your organs and improves your mental clarity and focus. By breathing mindfully and consciously, and slowing and deepening your breath, you can relax and ease anxiety and stress." You might be thinking, "I know how to breathe. I've been doing it my whole life." But deep breathing is a learned technique; it does not come naturally for most people.

When you're first learning how to do it, it's easier to do it lying down. Follow these steps:

1. Lie on your back with your legs extended and your arms comfortable at your sides.

2. Place one arm on your chest and the other on your abdomen.

3. Inhale slowly through your nose. You should feel your stomach expanding, which will cause the hand on your abdomen to rise. The hand on your chest shouldn't move much.

4. Exhale slowly, first through your nose and then through your mouth until the whole breath has been expelled.

If you're having a hard time getting it, that's okay; keep trying. Focus on making the hand on your abdomen rise as you inhale and fall as you exhale.

Strategy 6: Get Enough Sleep

Sleep is necessary in order to replenish your physical and emotional energies. The proper amount of sleep each night varies somewhat from person to person. Generally speaking, everyone needs around eight hours of sleep in a twenty-four-hour period. Some people require fewer hours, and others require more. Make no mistake, however: failure to get your required amount of sleep, whatever that might be, and not getting it night after night results in a condition called *sleep deprivation*. Those lost hours add up, and unless they are made up, you will experience the effects of sleep deprivation. Millions of people suffer from sleep deprivation in today's world of stressful jobs and hectic lifestyles. The results are that memory is impaired, reaction time slowed, and problem-solving skills and learning abilities are affected. How can you tell if you have sleep deprivation? If you fall asleep within five minutes of going to bed, doze off while watching TV or reading, and sleep in on weekends you are not getting enough sleep.

Insomnia is another sleep problem quite common in our culture today. Most of us have experienced some form of insomnia at one time or another. It is characterized by difficulty in falling asleep or waking up in the middle of the night and not being able to go back to sleep. Stress is a leading cause of insomnia, which can last from several days to several weeks. Usually, normal sleep returns once the stress is relieved. Utilizing some of the stress-reduction techniques discussed earlier should help in improving your sleep habits.

An important study done by Charles M. Morin at the Sleep Disorder Center at Laval University in Quebec offered some strategies for overcoming insomnia.

Here are some ideas to consider:

- Avoid caffeine in the late afternoon and evening, whether from coffee, soft drinks, chocolate, or other sources. Read your labels to find the hidden caffeine in what you are consuming.

- Avoid alcohol in the evening. It can disrupt your sleep later.

- Exercise regularly, at least three times a week, but avoid exercising three hours before going to sleep.

- Go to bed only when you feel sleepy. If you have trouble going to sleep, get up after twenty minutes and do something relaxing. Then, go back to bed and try again.

- If you have periods of wakefulness during the night, try to go to bed later than you normally do. After a few weeks, gradually increase your sleep time.

- Change your attitude about sleep. Do you become anxious if you don't fall asleep immediately? Do you fear you may have health problems? Identifying your fears and beliefs will help to de-emphasize them.

Travell and Simons (1983) and McKenzie (1997) also offer some suggestions for sound healthy sleeping:

- Avoid hard or bouncy pillows where the neck remains in a strained position all night. If you go on a trip, your comfortable home pillow should go along. Down-filled pillows are preferred, but not if you are allergic.

- If you sleep on your back, place a pillow under your knees.

- If you sleep on your side, bend at your hips and knees. Place a soft pillow between your knees. Also, it will help you to breathe easier and relax more if you have a pillow on which to rest your top arm.

- Try to avoid sleeping on your stomach. However, if you must, place pillows under the head, chest, and stomach.

- Have the appropriate pillows available as you change from one favorite position to another. Be creative. Find out what works for you.

- Sleep on a firm but not hard mattress.

- Roll up a beach towel and secure it at both ends with rubber bands. Stretch the towel out on the bed at waist level. This provides important lumbar support when you roll on either side.

- Begin your first minutes of going to sleep relaxing and doing deep breathing on your back. This helps to prepare you for a night of restful sleep.

Napping. Most of us could benefit from a little snooze, but unfortunately, our society does not allow for such luxuries during the average workday. If you are sleeping well at night, a daytime nap can restore energy and give you an important lift. If you are suffering from sleep deprivation, a short nap during the body's normal mid-afternoon slump can help make up for the deficit. Naps can make you sharper, healthier, and happier. A nap can be the difference between vigor and lethargy, success or failure. However, if you are having difficulty sleeping at night you may want to avoid napping until you overcome your nighttime sleep problems.

Just look at how far you have come in understanding TMJ disorder! I believe you are now beginning to see the important connection between your total body and the pain you are experiencing in your jaws. You have absorbed a lot of information, and it has not been easy. In Chapter 6 you will examine the issues of diet and exercise, and how they relate to TMJ disorder and your total well-being.

6

Evaluate and Improve Diet and Exercise Habits

A wellness plan can only succeed if attention is given to basic nutrition and exercise habits. Poor nutrition and lack of proper exercise are common problems in TMJ disorder sufferers. For years I have told patients, "You are what you eat. You cannot get high performance from your car on low-octane fuel. The same is true with you. What you put into your body, or fail to put in, profoundly affects the way you feel and your ability to resist infection and disease."

Early in my practice, I noticed a relationship between oral health and vitamin C deficiency in patients. Little research had been done back then on the effects of certain vitamins and minerals on our health. Studying the work of Adele Davis, Travell, and others made me a believer in the importance of obtaining the vitamins and minerals necessary to attain and maintain good health.

Diet and exercise always go hand in hand, so it's only natural to work on them together. Today, so much new information is coming out that it's easy to get confused. It's clear, however, that it's important to make an appraisal of your current diet. From there, you can identify the nutrients you're missing and utilize supplements or make changes in your diet. At the same time, you can start, or supplement, your own exercise regimen with the exercises provided in this chapter.

Vince, a twenty-five-year-old computer technician, was referred to me by his dentist on an emergency consultation for severe headaches that were determined to be caused by TMJ disorder. Vince reported the following symptoms: fatigues easily, cold hands and feet, dizziness, difficulty sleeping, muscle spasms, hand tremors, leg cramps, ringing in the ears, sinus problems, hearing difficulty, clicking and grating noises in the jaw joint, difficulty opening his mouth, pain while yawning, and pressure behind or around either eye. Vince was in so much pain that he suggested having all of his teeth removed.

When I asked Vince about his nutrition habits, he reported that he never ate at mealtime (he'd snack all day and before bed); mostly consumed coffee, soft drinks, white bread, refined sugar, canned vegetables, pastries, and TV dinners; ate no fruit or vegetables—frozen or fresh; and had been taking one multivitamin a day for the past four years.

He said the only exercise he got was walking up the stairs at work, and he tried to avoid doing that whenever possible. In addition Vince chewed gum, clenched his teeth, smoked cigarettes, and was overweight.

Although Vince needed a splint for a few months to ease the pain from clenching, we concentrated on his general nutrition and exercise program, both for his jaw and his general health. I referred him to a physical therapist. One week after starting to work with the physical therapist, he called me and said, "I told my physical therapist, 'You probably don't even realize what a difference you and Dr. Bob have made in my life, in less than a week.'"

Once Vince took charge of his wellness program, he was able to make significant changes in his lifestyle—starting with a diet and exercise program. He remains symptom-free.

Evaluate Your Eating Habits

First, review the Guide to Good Eating in figure 6.1 and ask yourself the following questions:

1. Do you eat foods from all five food groups every day?

2. Do you eat different foods from each food group every day?

Place a check mark next to each food that you eat every day and notice the number of servings per day that you need:

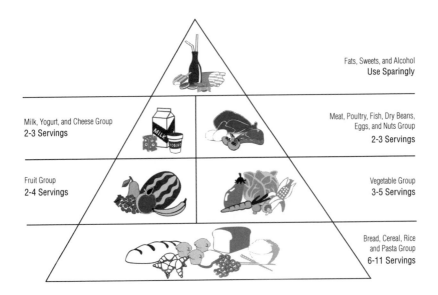

Figure 6.1. Guide to Good Eating

Source U.S. Department of Agriculture

Milk, etc. group (2–3 servings per day)

_____ Milk	_____ Cheese
_____ Cottage cheese	_____ Ice cream
_____ Frozen yogurt	_____ Ice milk
_____ Yogurt	

Meat, etc. group (2–3 servings per day)

_____ Cooked lean meat	_____ Cooked fish
_____ Cooked lean poultry	_____ Egg (1)
_____ Cooked dried peas	_____ Peanut butter (2 tbsp)
_____ Cooked dried beans	

Vegetable group (3–5 servings per day)

_____ Juice	_____ Raw leafy vegetables
_____ Cooked vegetable	_____ Potato

Fruit group (2–4 servings per day)

    ____ Juice   ____ Raw, canned, or cooked fruit

    ____ Apple, banana, orange, pear, cantaloupe, grapefruit

Grain group (6–11 servings per day)

    ____ Bread (whole grain)   ____ Cereal

    ____ English muffin   ____ Rice

    ____ Pasta   ____ Tortilla

As you study the Guide to Good Eating, decide if you are on target in all areas. Utilizing the columns in the following chart, list the food types you need more of, those you need less of, and those you are getting enough of on a daily basis.

I Need More	I Eat Too Much	I Eat Enough
Example:	Example:	Example:
Milk	*Fat*	*Fish*
Green vegetables	*Sweets*	*Poultry*
_____	_____	_____
_____	_____	_____
_____	_____	_____
_____	_____	_____
_____	_____	_____
_____	_____	_____
_____	_____	_____
_____	_____	_____
_____	_____	_____

Vitamins and Minerals

The following chart includes the vitamins and minerals that are essential for life, and the foods in which they are found. You will be able to determine for yourself where your deficiencies are. Remember, you need *all* of these vitamins and minerals *every day* for good health.

As you go through the list, write down all the foods that you eat on a regular basis next to each category. Don't worry if you find that you are repeating yourself. You will have a more complete picture of your total needs if you do it this way.

The Vitamin/Mineral Chart

Vitamins	Food Source	Foods You Eat Regularly
A is essential for normal vision, healthy mucous membranes, healthy skin, and resistance to infection. Vitamin A is an antioxidant. Beta carotene is converted into Vitamin A in humans.	Liver, fish liver; orange, deep yellow, and green leafy vegetables, such as carrots, pumpkin, winter squash, broccoli, spinach; eggs, cheese, butter, apricots, red or pink grapefruit.	_____ _____ _____
B₁, Thiamine is necessary for memory, emotional stability, and growth and functioning of nerve tissue.	Pork, beef, organ meats; whole wheat or enriched cereals; nuts, dried peas, and beans.	_____ _____ _____
B₂, Riboflavin is necessary for cellular growth.	Liver, milk products, dark green leafy vegetables, oysters, eggs, mushrooms, avocados, pastas, whole grains.	_____ _____ _____
B₃, Niacin is essential for energy production and the formation of red blood cells. Aids metabolism.	Organ meats, peanuts, poultry, muscle meats, legumes, whole grains, milk, eggs.	_____ _____ _____

Vitamins	Food Source	Foods You Eat Regularly
B₆, Pyridoxine plays a role in the multiplication of all cells and the production of red blood cells and cells of the immune system.	Bananas, soybeans, poultry, meats, organ meats, dried beans, peanuts, walnuts, avocado, salmon, whole grain cereals, wheat germ, egg yolk, broccoli, spinach, fresh tuna.	_____ _____ _____
B₁₂, Cyanocobalamin is essential for normal growth and the formation of healthy red blood cells. It is involved in maintaining a healthy nervous system.	Found only in animal products: meats; poultry; liver; seafood such as clams, oysters, salmon; egg yolks; milk, cheese, liver sausage (braunschweiger). (Vegetarians should consider supplementation if no animal products or by-products are consumed.)	_____ _____ _____
Folic Acid, Folacin is essential for DNA and RNA synthesis (carriers of genetic information), new cell growth (bone marrow) and the production of red blood cells.	Dark green leafy vegetables; organ meats such as chicken livers; kidney beans, asparagus, beets, cabbage, yeast, cauliflower, cantaloupe, wheat germ; and whole grain cereals and breads.	_____ _____ _____
C is essential for tooth and bone formation and healthy gums. It is involved in the immune response, resistance to infection and wound healing, and is an important antioxidant.	Citrus fruits and juices; tomatoes; sweet red, green and yellow peppers; potatoes, dark green vegetables; cabbage; cantaloupe and strawberries.	_____ _____ _____
D is necessary for normal formation of bones and teeth, aids in absorption of calcium and phosphorus.	Fortified milk, fish liver (cod liver oil); egg yolk, butter, oily fish (such as salmon, herring and sardines).	_____ _____

Vitamins	Food Source	Foods You Eat Regularly
E is an antioxidant and prevents the destruction of red blood cells.	Vegetable oils and seeds; wheat germ; margarine; green leafy vegetables; whole grain cereals; egg yolks; butter, milk fat; nuts and seeds.	_____ _____ _____
K assists in blood clotting.	Milk products.	_____ _____ _____
Pantothenic Acid is a B-vitamin involved in energy metabolism.	Liver, organ meats; fish; eggs; cheese; whole grain cereals and breads; avocado; cauliflower; green peas; dried beans; nuts; dates; sweet potatoes.	_____ _____ _____
Biotin is essential for the utilization of carbohydrates, proteins and fats.	Liver; organ meats; egg yolk; milk; yeast; whole grains; cauliflower; nuts; legumes.	_____ _____

Minerals	Food Source	Foods You Eat Regularly
Calcium is essential for bone and teeth formation, nerve impulse transmission, activating and relaxing smooth muscle, and blood clotting.	Dairy products (milk, cheese, yogurt); tofu, dark green leafy vegetables, canned fish with edible bones (such as sardines and salmon); nuts; dried peas and beans.	_____ _____ _____
Copper works with iron in red blood cell formation.	Shellfish; whole grain cereals; nuts; eggs; dried beans and peas; and dark green leafy vegetables.	_____ _____ _____

Minerals	Food Source	**Foods You Eat Regularly**
Iron is necessary for the formation of blood and the transportation of oxygen within the body.	Liver, organ meats, beef; dried fruits; peas and beans; dark green leafy vegetables; prune juice; farina; whole grain cereals and breads.	_____ _____ _____
Magnesium is essential for muscle relaxation and neuromuscular transmission and activity, necessary to a normal functioning heart. It prevents tooth decay by binding calcium to tooth enamel.	Nuts, legumes, whole grain cereals and breads, wheat germ; soybeans; dark green vegetables; milk; liver and beef.	_____ _____ _____
Phosphorus is essential to the growth, maintenance and repair of all cells. It works with calcium in building and maintaining strong bones and teeth.	Meat, soda pop, fish, poultry, eggs, cereals, legumes, processed foods.	_____ _____ _____
Potassium is the key nutrient inside the cell and plays a role in maintaining water balance, regulating muscle contractions and stimulating nerve transmission.	Potatoes, bananas, orange juice, apricots, cantaloupe, broccoli, meat, milk, peanut butter, avocado, lima beans, cabbage, spinach, mushrooms, tomatoes.	_____ _____ _____
Selenium is an antioxidant which protects cell membranes and enhances the activity of vitamin E.	Liver, kidney, meats; seafood (especially clams and oysters); whole grains; sunflower seeds; garlic.	_____ _____ _____

Minerals	Food Source	Foods You Eat Regularly
Zinc is essential for DNA and RNA synthesis, skin growth and wound healing.	Oysters, herring, clams, meat, chicken; milk, egg yolks; wheat germ; bran and nuts.	_____ _____ _____

Use the following chart to document your deficiencies:

Essential vitamins and minerals	I eat plenty of foods to get this nutrient every day	I eat some foods to get this nutrient every day	I rarely or never eat foods containing this nutrient
A			
B₁			
B₂			
B₃			
B₆			
B₁₂			
C			
D			
E			
K			
Folic Acid			
Pantothenic Acid			
Biotin			
Calcium			
Phosphorus			
Potassium			
Magnesium			

Essential vitamins and minerals	I eat plenty of foods to get this nutrient every day	I eat some foods to get this nutrient every day	I rarely or never eat foods containing this nutrient
Iron			
Zinc			
Copper			
Selenium			

What You Can Do to Improve Your Nutrition

You've made an honest appraisal of your present eating habits. Now you are in a position to evaluate just how good those habits are and to change them, if necessary. Before you rush out to buy supplements, consider these important points:

- Vitamins, minerals, and nutrients must be adequately supplied to your body each day.

- Foods should be the major supplier of these nutrients. They should be eaten in their natural state as much as possible. Fresh food is preferred over frozen. Frozen is better than canned. Unrefined foods should be used instead of refined.

- Each individual's needs are different. Use these guides as a way to increase your awareness of your particular eating needs and patterns and develop your own nutrition program accordingly. Sometimes there are health problems that require special consideration. Your age and state of health may also dictate a need for special supplements.

- All of us need vitamin E supplements because we cannot get enough from our diets. The recommended dose is 400 IU daily.

There are people who may need supplements for special reasons. In general, they include the following:

- People aged sixty-five or older whose bodies may not absorb the nutrients as well, or who do not eat properly. Frequently vitamins B_6, B_{12}, and D are recommended. Also additional calcium and vitamin D are needed for post-menopausal women. Often a multivitamin is preferred to help boost the immune system. Vitamin E has been confirmed as helpful in preventing cardiovascular disease.

- People who are on a strict weight-loss diet of one thousand calories a day may need a vitamin/mineral supplement.

- Smokers, because smoking reduces vitamin C levels and causes production of free radicals, those harmful substances that result from your body's cellular metabolism. Smokers need vitamin supplements that include adequate vitamin C and antioxidants.

- People who drink alcoholic beverages to excess have a need for additional nutrients. The alcohol has an adverse effect on the absorption, metabolization, and excretion of vitamins.

- Pregnant women or women who are breast feeding have a need for additional nutrients, especially folic acid, iron, and calcium.

- Vegetarians who eat no animal products or by-products may need additional B_{12}.

- People who have limited milk intake and very little exposure to the sun may need extra calcium and vitamin D.

What can you do with all this newfound information about yourself? It can certainly help you, and the health care professionals working with you, in assessing your individual needs. If you are not presently working with a health care professional, I would recommend discussing your needs with your local pharmacist or your county health nurses, who generally provide many public programs on nutrition and healthy living. There are also many good books on nutrition. One that I particularly like is Jean Carper's *Stop Aging Now!* (For information about this book refer to appendix A.) She says that the book is for anyone eighteen or older. Being on the far side of age eighteen, I find this book has particular significance for me. Whatever you do, I hope you will find ways to change and improve your general nutrition.

Adopt an Exercise Program

In chapter 2 we discussed exercises designed to improve the functioning of the jaw. Since the total body is involved in TMJ disorder, the Total Wellness Program must include exercises for all of the muscles of the body. In addition to benefiting your overall health, some exercises will also help prevent trigger points from returning. Before we go into the specific exercises, here are some general guidelines to remember:

- All muscles of the body should be stretched to their full range of motion every day, preferably by gentle, slow, and smooth movements. Start at your neck and make your way down to your feet.

- Muscles are designed to contract (tighten), relax, and be active. They were not meant to be immobilized for long periods of time; yet many people spend hours each day sitting behind a desk or computer. You can do three things to help in a situation like that:

  1. Get up and move around every twenty minutes

  2. Utilize correct posture when you are walking around to properly stretch and relax your muscles

  3. Use correct posture while sitting.

- Good posture prevents sustained contraction or prolonged shortening of muscles. For example, if you stand with your shoulders slouched and your head protruded, all of the weight is carried by the neck muscles. These muscles then tighten and must remain contracted in order to support the head. And so it goes throughout your body.

- Gentle, slow stretching of the muscles is preferred to any active program that exercises to the point of pain. You want to be able to feel the stretch, but not have it feel painful.

- Gentle stretching is the key to sustained relief from myofascial pain. After you accomplish that, you can increase your exercise regimen to include other forms of exercise that you enjoy. Do not try to combine them, however, until you are totally free from pain and feel comfortable with the stretching exercises as a part of your Total Wellness Program.

If you look at the various gentle stretching programs that are available today, you will find that most have roots in the ancient practice of yoga. I recommend a gentle yoga program, provided it is taught by a properly trained instructor. Read what James Baltzell, M.D., (1993) has to say about stretching, and about your muscles and joints. He also discusses the need for flexibility and establishing some rules about stretching. Regardless of what exercise program you adopt, these rules are important to remember.

Yoga is exercise, not a religion.

Yoga developed in the East many thousands of years ago before the advent of Nautilus and weight machines.... By placing the body in several different positions, a joint can be remobilized to become more flexible. This is called "doing yoga." Because these positions are not done in everyday life, they appear to be unusual. In fact, they are merely poses to stretch the joints in as many different positions as possible....

In the practice of yoga, there is a strengthening of all the muscle groups in the body in a gradual but steady manner. A large emphasis is placed on balance and symmetrical strengthening to avoid having one muscle group strong and another weak.... Strengthening the muscles results in more bone strength. This, in turn, is a way to retard the process of osteoporosis....

The concept of "no pain, no gain" does not apply in [yoga]. The purpose of the yoga exercise is to improve flexibility, not to cause pain. It is best to begin gently when starting stretching, as most people do not understand how much stretching is good for them. Each individual is responsible for how his/her body feels and, through doing the exercises, learns the optimum stretching for him/herself. The idea is to stretch the fiber around the joint without over-stretching and causing pain. There are two kinds of stretching: ballistic, or rapid stretching, and passive stretching. In yoga, passive stretching is performed, allowing the muscle fibers, ligaments, and tendons to stretch without going into spasm. This frequently takes from thirty seconds to five minutes, depending on the muscle group, and does require patience. However, during this holding time we learn how to relax and become more focused in our thinking. The following are some rules about muscle contraction and stretching:

Rule #1: No bouncing, as this causes the muscles to go into spasm.

Rule #2: Correct alignment of the body is extremely important.

Rule #3: Muscles shorten as the body moves. Stretching lengthens them. If we do not stretch, our muscles become shorter and harder, and painful and stressed. We become hunched-backed and even shorter as we age.

Rule #4: Muscles need to relax or they become deprived of oxygen. Stretching allows a rebound of relaxation and good flow of blood to the muscles.

Rule #5: Tight muscles hamper joints. Stretching promotes full range of motion. Otherwise, other body parts try to compensate and in the process deteriorate. Movement also promotes flow of synovial fluid, a lubricating fluid in the joints.

Rule #6: Tight muscles on one side of a joint mean weak muscles on the other side. Yoga balances so both sides work evenly. Many forms of exercise promote imbalance of the various muscle groups.

Rule #7: Tight muscles pull the body out of alignment and the joints out of alignment. This can cause uneven wear of the joints, particularly the knees and low back.

Rule #8: Stretching of the various ligaments around the joints allows the ligaments to be brought back into correct alignment.

The most important considerations right now are getting started on a plan that pleases you, finding a convenient time and place to do your exercises, and then faithfully doing them every day. The exercises I am suggesting can be done at home, without special equipment, at any convenient time, and won't cost you a cent. Let's take a look at them.

The Exercises

Caution: If you have health problems or have hurt your back previously, consult your health care professional before proceeding.

The following twenty exercises are simple stretching exercises that should become a lifetime habit, even when you increase your physical activity. You will find that each time you do the exercises you will be able to stretch just a little bit farther, lengthening the muscle and releasing any spasm that is there waiting to occur.

Start out by trying to do at least fifteen minutes of exercise each day. My instructions usually say "repeat five to ten times." This means start at five and work up to ten as your body feels able and willing. When you reach a maximum stretch, try to hold the position for at least ten seconds, and work up to thirty seconds. Concentrate on your abdominal breathing as you do your exercises. Always follow your exercise program with several minutes of relaxation and deep breathing.

1. Mountain Pose

The goal is to have this stance become a way of life. When correct posture becomes a habit, you will feel better all over. Stand evenly on both feet; toes pointed forward, feet together or slightly apart. Feel all four corners of each foot pressing down. If you rock forward and backward slightly, you will find your center of balance.

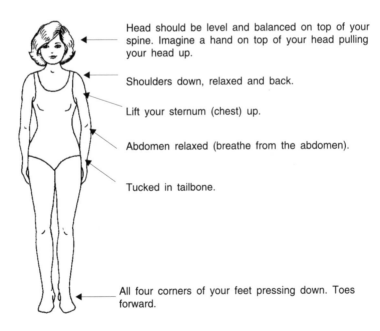

Head should be level and balanced on top of your spine. Imagine a hand on top of your head pulling your head up.

Shoulders down, relaxed and back.

Lift your sternum (chest) up.

Abdomen relaxed (breathe from the abdomen).

Tucked in tailbone.

All four corners of your feet pressing down. Toes forward.

Front View

Here's a side view of how to do the mountain pose correctly (in the middle) and incorrectly (on either side):

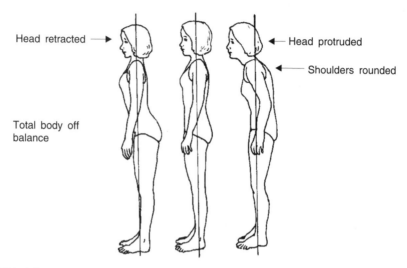

Head retracted →

← Head protruded

← Shoulders rounded

Total body off balance

Side View

The head weighs nine to thirteen pounds and is perched upon four small vertebrae. If the head is not properly positioned, it throws the entire body off balance, causing pain in various parts of the body.

2. Shoulder Shrug

Standing in mountain pose, pull your shoulders up as far as possible; hold for a few seconds, and release.

Do this exercise five to ten times.

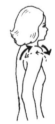

3. Shoulder Rolls

Standing in mountain pose, rotate your shoulders in circles, first going forward, and then rotating backward.

Do this exercise five to ten times in each direction, slowly.

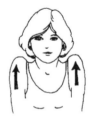

4. Upper Back Stretch

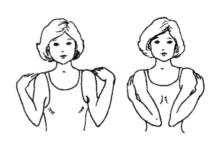

Standing in mountain pose, place your fingers on your shoulders. Then bring your elbows together in front of your chest. Keeping your fingers on your shoulders, make large circles with your arms, first rotating forward and then backward. Do this slowly and extend the stretch as much as possible.

Do this exercise five to ten times in each direction.

5. Arm Circles

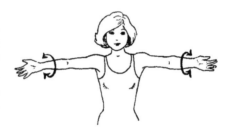

Standing in mountain pose, extend your arms to your sides at about shoulder height with your palms up. Make circles with your arms, first forward and then backward.

Do this exercise five to ten times in each direction.

6. Arm Stretch

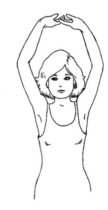

Standing in mountain pose, lock your fingers together in front of you, turn palms out and stretch your arms over your head or upward until you feel a slight stretch. Be sure to lift your arms slowly. Hold the stretch for several seconds.

Do this stretch five to ten times.

After you become comfortable during this stretch, you can add on to it by stretching from the waist to the right, then to the left.

7. Head and Neck Circles

Standing in mountain pose, gently rotate your head downward and around to the right in a large circle.

Do the circle five to ten times, change direction and repeat.

Do **not** do this if you feel pain.

Do not do this if fibromyalgia is a coexisting condition.

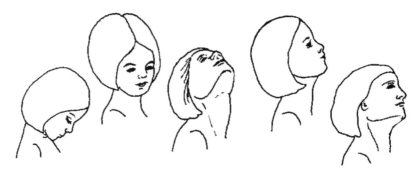

8. Hamstring Stretch

Using a chair for support, bend forward and clasp your hands around the back of the chair. Your legs should be straight, tailbone pointed to the ceiling, and your back straight. You should feel the stretch in the backs of your legs. Hold the stretch for fifteen to thirty seconds.

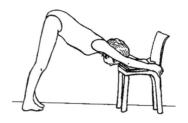

9. Back Stretch (Bend while sitting)

Sit on a chair with your feet touching the floor. Slowly and gently bend forward, letting your hands hang down toward the floor, until you feel a slight stretch in your back. Hold this pose for fifteen to thirty seconds.

Repeat three or four times.

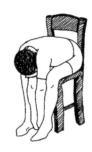

10. Pectoral Stretch

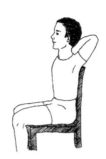

Sit on a chair and clasp your hands behind your head. Using the back of the chair for stability, stretch your arms back until you feel a gentle stretch in your chest. Hold for several seconds.

Repeat five to ten times.

The following exercises should be done on a firm surface, such as a floor or a bed with a firm mattress. If you're using a floor that has no carpeting, you can use an exercise mat or a towel if the floor is uncomfortable for you.

11. Pelvic Tilt

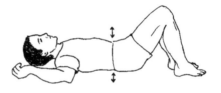

Lie on your back with your knees bent and feet on the floor. Slide your hand under your waist and you will see that it slips under easily. Now press your back *down* against the floor so your hand will not be able to slide under. Put your arms up next to your head and arch your back up, belly button up. Hold for several seconds, and repeat the down and up sequence.

This exercise will strengthen the abdominal muscles. Work up to ten times.

12. Modified Sit-up

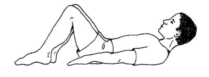

As you continue to lie on your back with your feet flat, slowly lift your head up to the count of two toward your knees until your shoulder blades no longer touch the ground. (Do not try to touch your knees.) Lower your head back to the ground to the count of two and then repeat the sequence five to ten times.

13. Knee to Chest

Lie on your back, knees bent, feet on floor. Grasp one leg behind the thigh and pull it toward your chest. Hold for several seconds. Do the same for the other leg. Then pull both legs up toward your chest and hold for several seconds.

Do this exercise five to ten times.

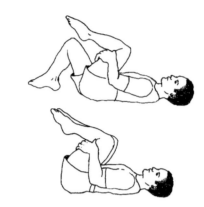

14. Flexion/Extension

While lying down on your back, knees bent, feet on floor, bend one leg up toward chest. Your arms should be at your sides supporting your body. Very slowly lower the leg until it extends full length and rests.

Do this two or three times with one leg and then do the same exercise using the other leg.

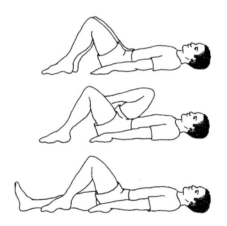

15. Hamstring Stretch
(Use a belt for this exercise.)

Lie flat, knees bent (1). Bend your right leg up toward chest (2). Place a belt around your right foot, then gently pull the leg straight up (3). Bring both of your legs down to rest position (4). Repeat with your left leg.

Repeat two or three times on each side.

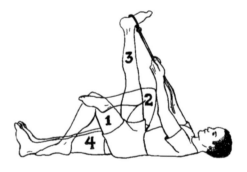

16. Spine Roll

Lie on your back, knees pulled up to your chest. Slowly roll to one side, keeping knees together. Rest in that position for several seconds, then roll to the other side.

Repeat three or four times.

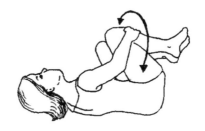

As an extension of this exercise, relax your shoulders and allow your upper body to be flat while your hips move to either side.

This exercise is especially relaxing when done on top of the bed before you go to sleep.

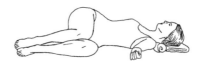

17. Cat Stretch

On your hands and knees, inhale as you arch your back and point your tailbone toward the ceiling. As you come up, exhale as you round your back, pulling in your abdomen and tucking your tailbone under. Repeat this sequence five to ten times.

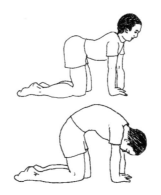

18. Kneeling Pectoral Stretch

After you do the cat stretch, extend your arms and stretch your body out as you lower yourself onto the backs of your legs.

Rest in this position and repeat a few times.

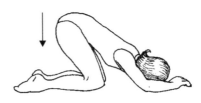

19. Legs up the Wall

With your head slightly supported, lie facing the wall with your bottom as close to the wall as possible. Stretch your legs up the wall, and rest for several minutes. You should feel a slight stretch in your hamstrings (back of the leg).

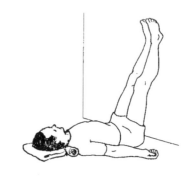

This exercise is restful and especially helpful if you are on your feet a lot during the day.

Keeping your knees straight, slide your feet apart, making a V with your legs, and feel the stretch in your inner thighs. Hold the position for a minute or more and increase the stretch. Repeat this part of the stretch a few times.

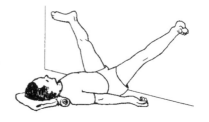

20. The Doorway Stretch

The doorway stretch is a good stretch for the chest, shoulders and back. Start in the doorway with one hand on either door jamb, about shoulder level.

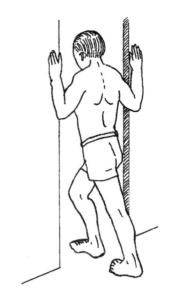

Step forward with your left foot and stretch your body forward. Hold this position for a few seconds. Then step your left foot back and step out with your right foot and hold the stretch for a few seconds.

Next, try it with your arms a little higher. Then try it with your arms a little lower, unless your physical therapist or doctor tells you not to.

It's good to do this stretch once or twice a day.

Congratulations on finishing part 1. You are now able to participate in your own wellness plan because you have the tools to understand the problem and make changes. You are in charge, and your health care professionals are there to assist you.

Read on to find important information on whiplash, fibromyalgia, and what to do if you need a splint. Part 2 is an important part of your education and understanding of TMJ disorder.

Part II

Other Considerations in Taking Control of TMJ

7

Whiplash and TMJ Disorder

Every year millions of people are involved in automobile accidents that result in whiplash injuries. Most victims seek medical help, either immediately or after a period of time has elapsed. Sometimes people go untreated, however, hoping the pain will just go away. Unfortunately, many of those people never fully recover and become so debilitated that they are unable to function either at home or at work. This should never happen. The major problem is simply this: health care professionals readily acknowledge that neck injuries have occurred in a whiplash-type accident (*cervical whiplash*), but all too frequently they fail to recognize that the jaw joint has been injured at the same time (*mandibular whiplash*). When the day comes that all health care professionals recognize the connection between these two injuries and treat both together, millions of people will recover and stay well.

There are many misconceptions about whiplash injuries, as well as disagreements among health care professionals. This chapter is intended to clear up some of the myths about whiplash and to provide knowledge for those who are suffering as a result of such an injury. You will be able to take a more active role in your healing once you have this information.

Judy, a thirty-year-old housewife, came to the office complaining of pain in her neck, shoulder, head, ears, chest, and back of her head. Six months earlier, she'd been involved in an automobile accident that resulted in whiplash.

As we went over her symptoms, Judy reported fatigue, swallowing problems, dizziness, cold hands and feet, and difficulty opening her mouth. She also complained of headaches, numbness in her fingers, pressure behind her eyes, hearing loss, frequent earaches, and a speech problem. Judy was deeply depressed as a result of the pain caused by the whiplash injury. She was totally incapacitated and unable to do many of the things so important in her life. She required professional counseling.

Judy was in extreme pain at our consultation appointment. She could only open her mouth about one-fourth of an inch. Routine clinical examination was out of the question. Any gentle attempt to check for head, neck, or shoulder trigger points was met with a knee-jerk reaction. She was hurting more than anyone I had ever examined. She needed a splint, but taking impressions to make the splint was impossible.

I had to improvise because she could only open wide enough to insert a warmed piece of dental wax between her back teeth. This served as a temporary splint to help relax the muscles that close the jaw. I encouraged her to make her own wax splint at home. I gave her some wax and suggested a few exercises for her to do. Ten days later she was able to open wide enough so I could take impressions to make the splint. She wore her splint full-time for about nine months. A properly constructed splint is, however, only part of the solution.

Why did Judy improve when others in a similar situation frequently do not? Judy worked hard to understand her total problem from head to toe and realized that progress would be slow. I explained to her that maximum medical results would take approximately two years. Judy had confidence in the professionals who were working on her behalf and participated in her treatment plan by faithfully doing her prescribed exercises and making some lifestyle changes.

Judy was referred to a physical therapist trained in managing patients who have been victims of whiplash. The therapist used a procedure called *myofascial release* (which you read about in chapter 3) in addition to more traditional methods. The progress Judy made was more than anyone could have expected. She saw a neurologist several times, and her improvement is well documented. She has completed physical therapy and is now using her splint only as a nighttime appliance. Judy's case was severe; yet many thousands of people have seen similar results with a little variation one way or another.

There are important lessons to be learned in this chapter that could make a real difference in your life. If you have *ever* been involved in a whiplash accident, this information could change your life.

What Is Whiplash?

When a person suffers a whiplash injury, the head and neck are unexpectedly or suddenly thrown very quickly in one direction and then rebounded in the opposite direction. Whiplash injuries occur in situations other than automobile accidents. They may occur as a result of sudden impact to the body, as in contact sports like football, hockey, or soccer. Falling, direct trauma to the skull, or even a sudden sneeze can cause a whiplash injury. The results are usually the same. For our purposes, however, we will be discussing whiplash from automobile accidents.

Statistics from the National Highway Traffic Safety Administration and the National Safety Council document that there are approximately 3.65 million whiplash injuries reported yearly from motor vehicle accidents. Whether the impact is from the rear, head-on, or from the side, severe neck injuries can result from such collisions. Garcia and Arrington (1996) reported that TMJ injuries (injuries to the jaw joint) occur in 87 to 97 percent of whiplash events.

All whiplash injuries are a little different because there are so many variables from accident to accident. In automobile whiplash we must consider

- What direction the driver was facing

- His/her age

- Amount of warning or state of preparedness

- The direction of the impact

- The speeds involved

If a seat belt was worn, there was some protection against the hyperextension aspect of the injury. Therefore, there are many symptoms and combinations of symptoms involved in these accidents. There is no "one size fits all" in whiplash.

Dr. Bruce H. Kinnie (1982) diagrammed what happens in various whiplash accidents:

In a rear-end collision (figure 7.1), the neck is thrown suddenly back beyond its normal range of motion (hyperextension) and then thrown suddenly forward (hyperflexion). Figure 7.2 shows the impact hyperextension in a rear-end collision has on the temporomandibular joint.

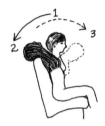

Figure 7.1. Collision from the Rear

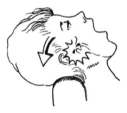

Figure 7.2. TMJ Injury when Hyperextension Occurs

In a head-on collision (figure 7.3), the head is thrown suddenly forward (hyperflexion) and then snaps back (hyperextension).

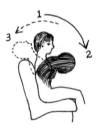

Figure 7.3. Head-on Collision

In a side collision (figure 7.4) the head (where a seat belt is not being worn), neck, and body are thrown towards the side of impact and then to the opposite side (that is, the head and neck are unexpectedly or suddenly thrown very quickly in one direction and rebound in the opposite direction).

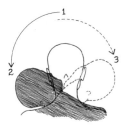

Figure 7.4. Collision from the Side

In the vast majority of whiplash injuries the damage is to the neck's ligaments, tendons, muscles, and vertebral alignment. In a small percentage of cases there is an actual bone fracture and spinal cord damage. Although it has been reported in the literature for many years, largely overlooked is the fact that in almost all traumatic whiplash injuries there is damage to the ligaments and muscles supporting the jaw joint as well. In any accident where the head is suddenly thrown back beyond its normal range (hyperextension), injuries to the temporomandibular joint can occur. And, according to Drs. Janet Travell and David Simons (1983), whiplash injuries can also activate certain trigger points.

Common Symptoms of Cervical Whiplash and Mandibular Whiplash

It's easy to see why there is confusion within the medical and dental professions on the whiplash/TMJ disorder connection. What follows are the most common symptoms reported by patients who either go to their doctor after a whiplash accident, or to their dentist for a TMJ disorder. The number of overlapping symptoms is startling; the reason, however, is not. Many of the same muscles, ligaments, and tendons are involved in both of these problems.

- Headache

- Neck pain

- Dizziness

- Pain deep in the ear and temporomandibular joint
- Pressure behind the eyes
- Tearing for no reason
- Earaches
- Hearing difficulty
- Ringing in the ears
- Fatigue
- Nervousness
- Numbness in the fingers
- Muscle spasms
- Muscle soreness
- Stiff neck
- Swallowing problems
- Depression

Here are symptoms of mandibular whiplash (TMJ disorder) *not* shared with cervical whiplash:

- Clicking, snapping, popping in your jaw
- Grating sounds of the jaw upon opening and closing
- Jaw deviates on opening and closing
- Inability to open the jaw fully
- Jaw locks open or shut
- Pain in the jaw joint
- Clenching

Common Myths about Whiplash

Until cervical whiplash and mandibular whiplash (TMJ disorder) are considered and treated together, I believe the confusion will continue. As a result, some common myths about whiplash will be perpetuated. Let's discuss them. First, I'll tell you what the myth is, and then I'll tell you why it's false.

Myth: You can not have a whiplash injury because the impact was so slight.

Truth: Injuries can result whether the impact is slight or severe.

Arthur C. Croft (1992) conducted extensive research on controlled studies that had been done of high-speed versus low-speed impacts resulting in whiplash injuries. The studies were done over a period of several years, in different locations in the United States and Canada, and by different researchers. Both human volunteers and crash dummies were tested at speeds ranging from seven to twenty miles per hour. Croft concluded that relatively low-speed collisions could produce significant soft tissue injury. Quite simply, this means that whiplash injuries can result whether the impact is slight or severe. Do not be put off by friends, professionals, or others who downplay your injury and pain because the accident appeared to be minor.

Myth: You can not have a whiplash injury because too much time has elapsed. If your present pain was related to your accident you would have had symptoms much earlier.

Truth: TMJ disorder symptoms can occur immediately, or can appear days, weeks, or even months after an accident has occurred.

A victim of a motor vehicle accident (MVA) whiplash injury usually consults first with a physician for complaints of headache, neck pain, and other musculoskeletal conditions. Treatment at this early stage frequently overlooks the temporomandibular joint entirely. Often the report says, "no organic cause for pain can be found." Yet TMJ disorder symptoms that dentists record months later were usually present at the time of the first medical exam. The Croft report (40) says,

> Both the cervical spine and the TM joint are especially vulnerable to injury regardless of the type of trauma, however trivial the injury may seem. Tissues in the neck and joint that have been stretched beyond their functioning capacity will result in various degrees of tearing. The sprains that occur do heal with the formation of less elastic scar tissue; however, the symptoms that focus on TMJ involvement are most often delayed and not identified.

If you recall in chapter 1, we discussed predisposing factors. These are things that happened to you long ago and set you up for problems later. These potential problems lie dormant until an event such as a whiplash injury occurs and brings them to the forefront. An early injury, jaw abnormality, or missing teeth are good examples of predisposing factors.

We've also already discussed perpetuating factors—things in your life that keep the problem going—that perhaps were not evident before the accident, but become a major problem afterward. Poor postural habits and how you react to stress and depression are good examples of perpetuating factors.

Errol Lader, D.D.S., author of *A Comprehensive Systems Manual* (1983) kindly adapted his "Sequential Effects of Cervical Trauma on the TMJ" model for this book to explain why a cervical whiplash injury can cause a TMJ disorder to develop at a later date:

Whiplash injury occurs.

↓

Sudden violent movement causes spasms in the muscles in the back of the neck.

↓

Muscles in the back of the neck shorten (contract) and the head moves slightly backward and upward.

↓

Specialized nerve cells in the neck muscles send messages to the brain: "There's trouble back here."

↓

The brain sends messages back to the neck muscles to correct backward/upward head position.

↓

To compensate, the head moves slightly forward to keep the eyes parallel to the ground. This causes increased tension in the front neck muscles, which attach to the lower jaw.

↓

Tension in the front neck muscles pull the lower jaw downward and backward.

↓

Now the upper and lower teeth do not align correctly and the "bite is off."

↓

Another message is sent to the brain: "Teeth are not aligning correctly."

↓

The brain sends messages back to the jaw muscles in an attempt to correct the bite.

↓

Tension increases in the jaw muscles.

↓

Constant increased tension causes spasms in the jaw muscles.

↓

The jaw muscle spasm causes stress in the temporomandibular joint.

↓

Stress in the temporomandibular joint causes TMJ disorder.

↓

The pain intensifies.

↓

The pain perpetuates spasms in the jaw muscles.

↓

The result is perpetuation of TMJ disorder.

Granted, this is a simplified version of the process that occurs in many whiplash injuries. But the process is accurate.

Myth: You can not have a whiplash injury because your X rays were normal.

Truth: Whiplash injuries are to the soft tissues and, unlike breaks in bones, are not evident on regular X rays.

How tragic that so many people are dismissed as malingerers or told, "It's all in your head," because nothing appears on an X ray.

Transcranial radiographs, panelipses, TMJ tomograms, and artho-grams do not record soft tissue injuries. They are effective in confirm-ing the diagnosis of internal derangement of the jaw joint, however (Garcia and Arrington 1996). While soft tissue injuries do show up on MRIs (magnetic resonance imaging), that does not mean that every patient should be given an MRI. They are very costly; so conservative treatment should be considered first in most cases.

The National Institute of Dental Research (NIDR) pamphlet for patients states that

> Regular dental X rays and TMJ X rays (transcranial radio-graphs) are not generally useful in diagnosing [TMJ disor-der]. Other X-ray techniques, such as arthrography (joint X rays using dye), magnetic resonance imaging (MRI), are usually needed only when the practitioner strongly sus-pects a condition such as arthritis or when significant pain persists over time and symptoms do not improve with treatment. Before undergoing any expensive diagnostic test it is always wise to get another independent opinion.

Let's accept the fact that these injuries do not readily appear on X rays, and get on with the matter of helping people get well.

Myth: You must be faking your pain, because the cervical collar you are wearing should make you feel better

Truth: While it is an accepted and appropriate treatment for the neck injury, the cervical collar often makes the TMJ injury worse.

Lader (1983) says,

> Some of the commonly prescribed treatment modalities that are currently used in the management of cervical inju-ries (i.e., cervical collars, cervical traction) can, in and of themselves, cause the development of temporomandibular joint disorders via the placement of direct mechanical pres-sure on the condyles of the TM joint complex resulting in compression of the vascularized joint component thus causing inflammation, and both local and referred pain.

If a cervical collar or cervical traction is prescribed for you, I would strongly recommend that you seek out a dentist knowledge-able in TMJ disorder and consider having a splint made. A splint will act as a spacer or shim between the teeth, thus offering protection to the injured joint while allowing healing to take place. A splint, when balanced properly, also aids in freeing trigger points and restoring normal muscle resting length. A word of caution, however: You notice I said *when balanced properly*. This is crucial to a splint being helpful to you. A splint that is not properly balanced can make the problem worse. In chapter 9, I discuss splints in more detail. Please read that chapter carefully before proceeding with splint therapy.

Challenge the Myths

Lader (1983, 87) found that

Due to the lack of recognition by the patient's health care provider(s) that traumatic injury to the neck can cause the manifold and seemingly unrelated symptoms of a TMJ [TMJ disorder] and chronic headache, many whiplash injury victims needlessly suffer with chronic intractable pain, and eventually manifest permanent degenerative changes in their temporomandibular joints.

If diagnosed early, before degenerative osteoarthritic changes become evident, TMJ Disorders can be treated with a predictably high degree of success. Once degenerative changes in the TMJ occur, however, some symptoms may remain on a permanent basis.

I have emphasized in this book that *knowledge is power*. It is important for you to have an understanding of what is happening to your body. Whiplash injury is complicated and contains many variables, and what one health care professional doesn't understand could have a lasting effect on you. No two people are alike; therefore, no two treatments will be the same. I would never second-guess the professionals working with you. This is truly a multidisciplinary problem, and almost always involves medicine, dentistry, physical therapy, and chiropractic. What I am suggesting, however, is that you challenge the myths and become a player on the team—the most important player at that. You will be able to direct the course of your treatment. You will have the ability to get well and stay well by using the information contained here.

8

Fibromyalgia and TMJ Disorder

Fibromyalgia syndrome (FMS) affects an estimated 2 to 5 percent of Americans (approximately 5 to 13 million people). It's difficult to pinpoint exactly how many people suffer from it because often it goes undiagnosed. Recent research has provided health care professionals with important new information about this complex and perplexing condition and how it relates to TMJ disorder. Since it is now estimated that 75 percent of fibromyalgia sufferers also have TMJ disorder, mostly in the form of myofascial pain, understanding both conditions is of the utmost importance. And since 18 percent of TMJ disorder patients develop fibromyalgia, health care professionals need to become familiar with the similarities in symptoms as well as the differences between these conditions. They also need to recognize that a person can have more than one condition at the same time. In fact, the following case study is about Jean, who had three conditions: cervical whiplash, mandibular whiplash (TMJ disorder), and fibromyalgia. Many people are misdiagnosed, fail to get well, and move from specialist to specialist because of this lack of knowledge.

All this new information and research can be pretty confusing. What I have tried to do is provide a simple overview of fibromyalgia to help you become aware of the connection between it and TMJ disorder and sort out the differences between them. If you feel that you may have a coexisting condition with your TMJ disorder, you should visit a specialist who understands rheumatic diseases. A *rheumatic dis-*

ease or disorder is any of several pathological conditions of muscles, tendons, joints, bones, or nerves characterized by discomfort and disability.

Jean, a fifty-year-old rural mail carrier, was referred to me by a federal medical nurse who worked with people receiving worker's compensation. Two and a half months earlier, Jean had been involved in a rear-end automobile accident that had resulted in whiplash injuries. She complained of "pain all over" and said she felt "tired, cranky, and miserable."

As we went over her symptoms, Jean reported fatigue, swallowing problems, cold hands, memory loss, dizziness, emotional upsets, difficulty sleeping, muscle spasms, leg cramps, muscle soreness, frequent nose bleeds, clicking in the jaw joint, frequent earaches, hearing difficulty and frequent urination. She reported pain in all parts of her face, head, neck, shoulders, back, legs, and feet.

Jean had been evaluated by four physicians. The first physician prescribed Ibuprofin. The second physician prescribed 600 mg Motrin every three hours and 600 mg Tylenol every three hours. It proved to be too much for Jean, so she stopped taking the medicine and went to a neurologist. The neurologist attributed her problem to old age and told her to take the medicine her other physician had prescribed. She decided to try yet another physician, who diagnosed whiplash and took her off all medications. He suspected fibromyalgia. When she was referred to me, she was receiving counseling and physical therapy. However, she felt that her condition was worsening. Why was Jean getting worse? She was getting worse because she had more than one problem. In addition to the cervical whiplash from the auto accident, she had mandibular whiplash as well (see chapter 7). And, as her fourth physician found, her total body symptoms indicated the presence of a third problem: fibromyalgia.

Jean was lucky to have found a team of professionals who could work together, understand the complexity of the problem, believe in her, and accept her as a key player on the team. Here are the members of her team:

- A federal medical nurse, assigned by Worker's Compensation to coordinate all of Jean's health care professionals

- A physician who understood fibromyalgia syndrome

- A dentist who was knowledgeable about TMJ disorder and whiplash

- A physical therapist trained in myofascial release

- A rehabilitation counselor who was a clinical psychologist

- Jean, who was willing to listen, make appropriate behavioral changes, and recognize her limitations then and in the future

Jean understood that it would take about two years for her to achieve maximum medical improvement. She was motivated to get well and to be able to work up to her potential. She learned to make adjustments in her lifestyle and has made significant progress. She had setbacks following a four-hundred-mile driving trip to Chicago, and two six-hour round-trip drives for examinations by post office orthopedic specialists. Even though she stopped to stretch and rest at one-hour intervals during each trip, she regressed for several days each time.

What Is Fibromyalgia?

Fibromyalgia syndrome (FMS) is a painful, debilitating condition that affects many areas of the body and causes fatigue. Women suffer from FMS more than men do. Despite the fact that millions of Americans have FMS, it was only officially recognized as an illness by the American Medical Association in 1987. According to Starlanyl and Copeland (1996, 8),

> Now, nearly ten years later, it is still, unfortunately, too often dismissed as the "newest fad disease," and most physicians still lack the diagnostic skills needed to differentiate it from other chronic pain conditions. In fact, until recently, it was rare to find a doctor who had even heard of FMS as a "real" condition, and very few doctors have received any substantial training in treating the syndrome. ... The average FMS patient suffers for five years and spends thousands of dollars on medical bills before receiving an accurate diagnosis.

Causes of FMS

What causes FMS is yet to be determined. Some researchers blame an injury or trauma that affects the central nervous system. In a study of 161 patients who had been injured, 102 had soft tissue injuries to the neck (90 percent having classic whiplash), and 59 patients had leg fractures. More than 20 percent of the patients with neck injuries developed fibromyalgia, whereas only 1.7 percent of the patients with leg fractures developed fibromyalgia (Bennett 1997). Others believe that stress or emotional trauma is instrumental in the onset of FMS. Those who suffer from it, however, are less concerned about how they got it and more concerned about how to treat it.

FMS Symptoms

Symptoms of FMS are many and varied, which is part of the reason physicians have such a difficult time diagnosing it. Common symptoms include the following:

- Motor coordination problems (body imbalance)
- Irritable bowel syndrome
- Irritable bladder syndrome
- Rapid heartbeat
- Headaches
- Sensitivity to smells, sounds, lights, and vibrations
- Cold intolerance
- Dry eyes
- Extreme, severe foot cramps
- Unexplained widespread pain or ache
- Restless legs (constantly moving, day and/or night)
- Generalized morning stiffness
- Nonrefreshing sleep
- Multiple tender points
- Atypical patterns of numbness and tingling
- Inability to exercise and complaints of weakness
- Periods of mental confusion and/or forgetfulness

Diagnosing FMS

In order to be diagnosed with FMS, you must have eleven or more of the eighteen tender points indicated in figure 8.1. Your tender points must also be present in all four quadrants of the body (upper right and left, lower right and left). *Tender points* are like trigger points in that they hurt when they are pressed; but, they *do not* refer pain to other parts of the body. When checking for tender points, press on the spot with your thumb. Use enough pressure to make the tip of your nail turn white. You can check yourself using the dots on figure 8.1 and the following guide. This information is taken from Starlanyl and Copeland's book, *Fibromyalgia & Chronic Myofascial Pain Syndrome* (1996, 10–11).

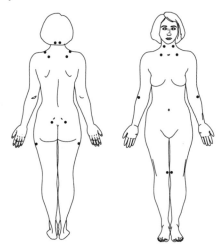

Figure 8.1. Location of Tender Points

On the *back* side of your body, tender points are present in the following patterns:

- Along the spine in the neck, where the head and neck meet

- On the upper line of the shoulder, a little less than halfway from the shoulder to the neck

- Three finger widths, on a diagonal, inward from the last point

- On the back fairly close to the "dimples" above the buttocks, a little less than halfway in toward the spine

- Below the buttocks, very close to the outer edge of the thigh, about a finger width

On the *front* side of your body, tender points are present in the following patterns:

- On the neck, just above inner edge of the collarbone

- On the neck, a little further out from the last points, about four fingers down

- On the inner (palm) side of the lower arm, about three finger widths below the elbow crease

- On the inner side of the knee, in the "fat pad"

If your symptoms indicate that you may have FMS, look for a physician knowledgeable in the field of rheumatology and check it out.

Treatment for FMS

While there is no cure for FMS, sufferers can ease the pain and discomfort through a variety of treatments. Treatment for FMS usually includes some combination of patient education, physical therapy, counseling, medication, nutritional supplements, stress reduction techniques, and a low-impact exercise program.

Fibromyalgia and TMJ Disorder: The Differences and Similarities

With the help of Starlanyl and Copeland (1996) and Slavkin (1997), I have developed a comparison chart of TMJ disorder and FMS to help sort out the differences and similarities between these complex and confusing disorders.

TMJ disorder	FMS
Chronic pain affecting women more than men; decrease in prevalence with age	Chronic pain affecting women more than men; increase in prevalence with age
18.4 percent of TMJ disorder patients also have FMS	75 percent of FMS patients also have TMJ disorder
Both nerves and muscles are affected	The chemical composition of the body is out of balance
Pain is referred from myofascial trigger points to specific areas, usually in the head, neck, and shoulders	Eleven to eighteen tender points throughout the body, and widespread pain (sometimes myofascial trigger points are present also)
Specific pain in specific areas	Body wide, diffuse achiness

Here's a list of symptoms common to both TMJ disorder and FMS to help you see why there is confusion within the medical and dental professions when it comes to diagnosing and treating these patients:

- Persistent fatigue
- Shortness of breath
- Headaches
- Knee, leg, and foot pain
- Numbness in fingers
- Osteoarthritis
- Eye pain
- Anxiety and depression
- Earaches
- Unexplained toothaches
- Hearing difficulty
- Dizziness (vertigo)
- Ringing in the ears

Common TMJ disorder symptoms not usually found in FMS patients include the following:

- Clicking, snapping, popping noises in the jaw joint
- Grating sounds and deviation of the jaw upon opening and closing
- Jaw locking open or shut
- Pain in the jaw joint
- Inability to open the jaw fully
- Clenching

If You Have Both Conditions

If you are experiencing symptoms of fibromyalgia in addition to your TMJ disorder symptoms, I recommend reading Starlanyl and Copeland's book and consulting with your physician or dentist before you proceed further into treatment. The commingling of symptoms makes proper diagnosis difficult and could explain why a particular treatment you are receiving is not helping. However, since this is a medical problem, dentists should be cautious about making any judgments on the FMS connection. FMS is a complicated illness, and other conditions coexist with it that require careful clinical diagnosis from a competent specialist. A true team approach is necessary for successful management of these problems. We must hope that Starlanyl and Copeland's book gets into the hands of the medical profession quickly so that health care professionals and concerned people like you will be able to find knowledgeable physicians. Regardless of which problem you may have, or if you have both of them, The Total Wellness Program can enhance your recovery.

9

Splints

If you have been told you need to wear a splint in your mouth, or if one has already been made for you, you need to understand what that appliance is supposed to do for you. If your splint is not constructed or balanced properly, it can do more harm than good. I've seen too many situations where the splint was improperly designed or balanced, the patient's symptoms worsened, and the dentist referred the patient for surgery because there didn't appear to be any other choice. This should *never* happen. The good news is that you can play a key role in attaining successful treatment using a splint if you have the right information, understand what the splint is supposed to do, and know how it should feel.

Gary, a fifty-four-year-old carpenter with a history of work-related injuries, was referred to me by his dentist for a TMJ consultation. His chief complaint was pain, sometimes severe, on the right side of his jaw. He was not able to open his mouth very wide without pain. Eating was difficult for him.

As we went over his symptoms, Gary reported fatigue, swallowing problems, muscle spasms and soreness in his legs (leg cramps). He also reported dizziness, sinus problems, numbness in his fingers, headaches, hearing difficulty, and difficulty sleeping. His jaw muscles were usually sore when he woke up in the morning. He was clenching and had noticed clicking and grating noises in his temporomandibular joint. He also reported upper and lower backaches. He'd had back surgeries in 1974 and 1991.

Gary was typical of many TMJ disorder patients. He had two problems, or diagnoses, as we dentists call them: myofascial pain in the head and neck, and internal derangement of the temporomandibular joint.

I prescribed a splint for Gary and introduced him to the Total Wellness Program. Figure 9.1 shows the type of splint I used on Gary. Figure 9.2 shows Gary's profile before treatment, and then after, with the appliance in place. You will note the change and improvement in his profile when the jaw reached its optimum position with the help of the splint.

There are many different types of splints used in TMJ therapy. Each dentist has his or her favorite one and reasons why that's the case. I do not intend to engage in a debate about which splint is best; such controversy is not helpful to you. More important is that not all dentists know how to balance splints correctly, and this is where the problems arise.

What Are Splints?

Splints are removable plastic bite-plates that fit over either the upper or lower teeth. Some splints cover all of the teeth, while others cover only the lower back teeth. They are sometimes called *orthotics* or *mandibular orthopedic repositioning appliances*. There are differences of opinion among dentists as to which type of splint is best. Regardless of the type, however, all splints used in TMJ disorder treatment are supposed to

- Help alleviate the painful symptoms of TMJ disorder

- Allow for healing to take place in the jaw joint

- Aid in breaking the habit of clenching

- Allow the lower jaw to rotate downward and forward, easing the problem that exists in the temporomandibular joint

- Give the back teeth freedom to move if they need to, allowing the condyles to stabilize in a more comfortable, natural position at the completion of treatment

It's important to understand that your teeth are not set in stone, so to speak; they can move from day to day, or week to week. Clenching and other harmful habits can hamper this movement. Splints, as well as exercises that relax the mandible, allow teeth to move the way they need to.

Who Needs a Splint?

In chapter 1 you read about causes and contributing factors of TMJ disorder and learned that the vast majority of TMJ disorder patients have two problems:

1. *Myofascial pain in the head and neck area, as a result of trigger points that refer pain.*

2. *Internal derangement of the temporomandibular joint due to any or all of the following reasons:*

    • A poor bite (malocclusion), which can be a result of skeletal discrepancies, missing teeth, worn-out dentures that allow the jaw to overclose, any opening of the jaw for a prolonged period, or even a big yawn

    • Any traumatic injury to the head, face, jaw or neck (The event need not be recent, and the injury could be considered minor, as in a minor whiplash accident.)

    • Bad postural habits or oral habits that promote clenching, such as chewing gum, having poor eating habits, and engaging in activities that strain the neck or back

Myofascial pain is by far the most common form of TMJ disorder, and is treatable by following the Total Wellness Program. Splints are not required for this type of problem. When internal derangement is part of the diagnosis, often a splint is needed to aid in the healing process. Remember that internal derangement means that the disc between where the lower jaw (condyle) and the upper jaw connect is displaced. See figure 1.1 if you need to refresh your memory. Maintaining a critical 3-millimeter joint space is the objective of successful treatment.

How a Splint Works

Regardless of the type of splint prescribed for you, the important thing for you to remember is that the splint must be positioned properly in order to help. Proper position is not universal and must be determined for each individual. The jaw must be in the optimum position (called *physiological rest position*) for each patient—that is, where the jaw functions best. You will be able to feel the jaw muscles relax when the splint is properly adjusted. Although it might feel strange at first, it should feel comfortable to you. If the splint holds the jaw in a tense or awkward position, the muscles will contract and eventually go into spasm. As a result, that position will then become habitual, and pain will persist.

The splint that I like best and have used with TMJ disorder patients for the past twenty years is called a *mandibular orthopedic repositioning appliance*, or *MORA* (see figure 9.1). It covers the lower back teeth only. Often I uncover the back molars on both sides (if they are present) to allow for eruption of the second molars. A tooth tends to erupt until it contacts the opposing tooth. If this is allowed to happen, the condyle is no longer forced up and back. Instead, the condyle moves downward and slightly forward, leaving room for the disc to return to its desired position, on top of the condyle. This position, if allowed, will become stable. If clenching continues, it will not stabilize.

The MORA, according to its designer, Dr. Harold Gelb, has many advantages:

- It can be constructed quickly and is easy to correct or adjust.

- It provides the patient with comfort in the shortest period of time.

- Jaw clicks disappear.

- The facial profile will improve.

- The procedure is reversible.

- The appliance can be discarded, if it's not effective, without damaging the teeth.

Figure 9.2 shows the profile of Gary, the TMJ disorder patient you read about at the beginning of this chapter. Note the improvement in the facial profile. The lower jaw was brought down and forward, eliminating TMJ disorder symptoms and improving his bite as well as his profile.

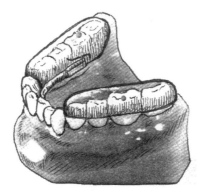

Figure 9.1. The MORA

Adapted from a photo provided by Johns Dental Laboratories, Terre Haute, Ind.

Once the best jaw position has been determined, and a splint is being used properly, healing in the temporomandibular joint will begin. The prescribed exercises and behavioral modification changes contained in the Total Wellness Program will then determine the success or failure of treatment. Once you have participated in the Total Wellness Program, and are showing significant progress, I encourage you to go without the splint as often as possible, using it mainly as a nighttime appliance. Before this can happen, however, the prescribed exercises and behavioral changes must become healthy habits.

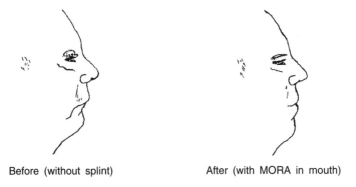

Before (without splint)   After (with MORA in mouth)

Figure 9.2. Gary's Profile (Adapted from actual photos)

When you're using your splint, remember that the condyles must be allowed to function in a pain-free position (this position will permit the disc to function where it was intended). During sleep, the appliance shouldn't allow the mandible (jaw) to move backward or to the side. It should also allow the posterior teeth to erupt. Since the desired outcome is to have the condyles functioning in a pain-free position, orthodontic or prosthetic treatment may need to be considered as a permanent solution. That means you may have to move teeth to achieve a more desired result both functionally as well as aesthetically. Prosthetic treatment means using crowns, bridges, or partial dentures in cases where teeth are missing (Witzig 1994).

Your dentist may be using a splint that is different from the one I have described. This is fine if you are showing progress, and your symptoms are diminishing. Fricton (1988) suggests that splints are more effective in combination with other treatments such as physical therapy, behavioral modification, stress management and nutritional counseling.

Splints frequently used for TMJ disorder are called

- *Upper (maxillary) flat bite plane splints*

- *Lower repositioning splints* (like the MORA), which allow back molars to erupt

- *Anterior bite planes,* which permit bicuspids (teeth with two cusps) and molars to erupt

I asked a colleague, William E. Stein, for his thoughts on functional appliances and TMJ disorder; here is what he had to say:

In certain cases of TMJ disorder where malformation of the teeth or jaws is the main problem, the dentist may use "Functional Orthopedic Appliances" instead of the usual splint. Functional appliances come in many shapes and designs but all have the advantage of correcting the malformation while serving as a "splint," thus correcting the main cause of the problem while keeping the patient out of pain and therefore saving time and expense, not to mention the agony of TMJ disorder. Functional appliances are effective in the gross correction of malformation, but "braces" may be needed to put the finishing touches on the case; however, functional appliances do drastically shorten the amount of time "braces" need to be worn.

Before you make a final decision on what is best for you, consider what Dr. Charles S. Greene, Director of Orofacial Pain Studies, University of Illinois College of Dentistry (1992, 45) says about them:

- Splints are both the best thing and the worst thing ever to appear in the TMJ disorder field. In one form or another, splints have been around for more than 50 years. Certainly many thousands of patients have been helped by their use. Unfortunately, the potential for serious negative outcomes also is very high for splints, because they can produce irreversible occlusal and jaw position changes.

- Most modern authorities recommend splint therapy as a temporary measure with the therapeutic goals being relaxation of muscles, altering joint loading (reducing forces that can be damaging to the various tissues that make up the temporomandinular joint), and general relief of symptoms.

- The proper rule of thumb for the use of splints is: "Do no harm."

You have just completed a short course on splint therapy. Keep in mind that a splint will not solve your TMJ problem on its own. You have to stick with the Total Wellness Program in order to achieve maximum benefits.

10

Helpful Therapies: Treatment Options to Consider

A number of other therapies have proven to be effective in treating patients with TMJ disorder. The following are brief summaries of the ones that many of my patients have tried and found helpful, so I feel comfortable recommending them to you. These are by no means the only treatment options to consider. There may be other options that will be suggested by your health care professionals. You will be the final judge of what works best for you. Other options you can consider using in conjunction with the Total Wellness Program include the following:

- Physical therapy—for a wide range of helpful treatments

- Myofascial Release—when pain is severe and other treatments are too strenuous

- Myotherapy—can be done at home

- Chiropractic—make sure the chiropractor understands myofascial trigger points

- Gentle yoga—as part of a lifetime exercise program

- Biofeedback—if pain is severe and other treatments fail

- Podiatry treatment—if you discover that problems in your feet are contributing to your condition

Physical Therapy

The physical therapist plays a central role in treating patients with TMJ disorder. TMJ problems most often involve the total body, in addition to the head, neck, shoulders, and jaw, so the many treatment options offered by physical therapists can be helpful. In chapter 2 you read about the major jaw exercises recommended by Mariano Rocabado, world-renowned physical therapist. The following are additional treatments available through a physical therapy clinic.

If you are in acute pain, the following treatments may be prescribed:

- Ice—to reduce inflammation

- Myofascial Release—to release trigger points in affected muscles

- Joint mobilization exercises—to improve joint range of motion

- Pulsed ultrasound—painless soundwaves directed at the painful area to reduce inflammation and increase circulation

- Electrical stimulation—gentle, painless electrical impulses directed at tense muscles to break up the spasm and increase circulation

- Ionophoresis—the use of electrical stimulation that produces deep heat to expedite therapy

- Exercises—to restore muscle length of contracted muscles

If your pain is chronic, a physical therapist may use the following treatments:

- Heat, moist or dry—to release muscle spasms and increase circulation

- Myofascial Release

- Massage—to relax tight muscles and improve circulation

- Joint mobilization exercises

- Ultrasound—painless non-pulsating sound waves directed to the affected area to reduce swelling and inflammation and increase circulation

- Exercises

- Referral for counseling when needed

In addition to these treatments, physical therapists evaluate the total body. They may provide instructions on any of the following:

- Stabilization exercises to promote strength and flexibility

- Reestablishment of normal posture

- Instruction on diaphragmatic (deep) breathing

- Relaxation and stress management techniques

Myofascial Release

You learned about the importance of fascia in chapter 1. Remember that *myo* refers to muscle. *Fascia,* according to Barnes, "is a tough connective tissue which spreads throughout the body in a three-dimensional web from head to foot without interruption. The fascia surrounds every muscle, bone, nerve, blood vessel and organ of the body all the way down to the cellular level. Therefore malfunction of the fascia system due to trauma, posture, or inflammation can create the binding down of the fascia resulting in abnormal pressure on nerves, muscles, bones or organs."

Because the structure of fascia is three-dimensional, when it malfunctions, an enormous pressure results (approximately 2000 pounds per square inch) and creates pain. Only Myofascial Release procedures release that pressure.

Myofascial Release (MFR) is a relatively new addition to the list of helpful therapies utilized by physical therapists, physicians, dentists, chiropractors and others in treating TMJ disorders. John Barnes, P.T., who developed MFR, defines it as follows:

Myofascial Release is generally an extremely mild and gentle stretching that has a profound effect upon the body tissues. Myofascial Release is a whole body "hands on" approach to the evaluation and treatment of the human structure. The therapist is taught to evaluate the fascial system to determine where the fascial restrictions lie. He or she will apply gentle pressure into the direction of the restriction.

MFR is one of the best forms of therapy for patients with fibromyalgia, whiplash, or TMJ disorder. It also has a strong emotional component. Therapists are trained to recognize depression in their patients and make appropriate referrals for counseling when necessary.

Myotherapy

Myotherapy is a system of erasing muscular pain that combines applying pressure to myofascial trigger points, gentle massage, and specific exercises to relieve pain, release tension, and improve range of motion and circulation. The therapy (which was also discussed in chapter 3) was developed by Bonnie Prudden and is described in detail in her book *Pain Erasure: The Bonnie Prudden Way*. The book provides a handy guide to locating trigger points, deactivating them with seven seconds of pressure, and preventing their return by specific exercise. Some physical therapists and chiropractors now utilize Myotherapy, and many myotherapists are trained and practicing throughout the country. To locate one, you can contact Bonnie Prudden Pain Erasure Clinic, 7800 E. Speedway, Tucson, AZ 85710. If you want to try to do it yourself, there are complete instructions for the lay person in Prudden's book.

Chiropractic

Chiropractic is a system of therapy in which disease is considered the result of abnormal function of the nervous system. In researching the field of chiropractic, I asked my colleague, Dr. Dale Hultgren, D.C., of Crosslake, Minnesota, for his insights on the subject. Here's what he said:

> D. D. Palmer, the founder of chiropractic over a century ago, theorized that an irritation to the nervous system could result in pain, numbness, spasm, paralysis, or disruption of the function of the different parts of the body. Conventional science has proven his hypothesis correct. It is no longer considered quackery to accept the fact that the brain and nervous system control the function of the entire

body. Chiropractic emphasizes the maintenance of health by adjusting spinal misalignments that irritate the nerves.

As with any profession, chiropractic is constantly improving and modifying its methods of treatment. However, the primary hypothesis of the nervous system controlling function of the body, that is, that any interference to the nervous system may cause malfunction of the body, is still the same as it was back in 1895. What has changed is the method of finding and correcting the misalignments of the spine. Within the profession there are two schools of thought and practice: those who hold to the original practice of locating and adjusting the spine by hands only, and those who utilize physiotherapy methods to aid in correcting the "pinched nerves." In years past these two factions were adamantly in opposition to each other. Today there is less distinction between the two, and more acceptance of each other's methods.

Chiropractors who have studied myofascial pain can be a great help in facilitating healing in people with myofascial trigger points. Chiropractors are knowledgeable about the entire body and know how to search out and find muscular trigger points in all parts of the body. They may use soft tissue manipulation to eliminate the trigger points and relax the muscle. Some use trigger-point therapy, or Myotherapy, to relax the contracted muscles. Many of the treatments discussed in the Physical Therapy section are employed by chiropractors, especially the use of ice or heat, electrical stimulation, ultrasound, and joint adjustment when needed.

Gentle Yoga

There are many forms of yoga. For that reason I am stressing gentle yoga and recommending it as the preferred therapy for people with TMJ Disorder. *Hatha yoga* is a series of exercises that are designed to keep joints flexible and stretch the muscles and tendons. A complete set of exercises takes each joint through a full range of movement and stretches all the major muscle groups. Proper breathing techniques are taught at the same time.

The exercises are referred to as *postures,* or *poses,* because the participant is encouraged to hold a position for up to several minutes to receive maximum benefit from the stretch. Because it is so important to do each exercise correctly, I encourage you to seek out a qualified instructor in the beginning so that you learn the proper technique.

You do not have to be in peak physical condition to benefit from yoga. There is no age limit, and you work at your own pace. You will find that you make progress each time you gently stretch. Yoga tends to "reverse" many of the symptoms of ill health and aging. You will find a more complete explanation of yoga in chapter 6.

Biofeedback

Biofeedback is a procedure where a therapist attaches an electronic monitoring device to your body in order to measure such things as blood pressure, heart rate, and jaw tension—things you didn't know you could influence. The treatment involves teaching relaxation techniques as well as helping the patient control those physiologic activities. Biofeedback can be helpful for TMJ disorder because it not only reinforces the relaxation response, but also provides information to patients about the negative impact of habits such as clenching and bruxing on muscle activity.

If you'd like more information, contact Biofeedback Certification Institute of America, 10200 West 44th Ave., Suite 304, Wheat Ridge, CO 80033.

Podiatry Treatment

A number of years ago, Drs. Travell and Simons made me a true believer in the importance of the feet to TMJ disorder. They were featured speakers at a symposium entitled "Myofascial Pain Dysfunction: Lower Back and Limbs." How strange that a dentist would be concerned about the legs and feet. However, a number of dentists, I found out, had achieved success in the treatment of TMJ disorder when problems in the lower limbs had been recognized and treated. This meeting was a major breakthrough for me in understanding and treating the total patient. This knowledge resulted in a much higher success rate in treatment for my patients.

Further study of foot problems, and their relationship to TMJ disorder, led me to Howard J. Dananberg, a New Hampshire–based podiatrist and leading researcher in the study of feet and gait analysis. He had this to say: "Some aches and pains, such as corns, bunions, fallen arches, and spurs are easily recognizable as problems directly associated with foot abuse or malaise. Other ailments caused by the way we walk are not so readily apparent as foot problems." For instance, he points out, that "some knee, hip, and back pain, arthritis, and TMJ disorder can frequently be traced to *functional hallux limitus (FHL)*. This is a foot problem characterized by failure of the hinge joint, located between the toe and the ball of the foot, to flex at the right moment when you are taking a step."

The following chart developed by Dr. Dananberg is a concise summary of what occurs when you have a faulty walk, or gait. If you are experiencing any of the problems described by Dr. Danenberg, you may want to consult a podiatrist.

Style of Gait	Indications	Potential Problems
Normal		
Heel-toe gait. Power stride with good balance and ease of step. Feet pointed straight or slightly out.	Even wear on shoes	Little if any complaints of poor posture or back/leg soreness.
Toe-Out		
Duck toe gait that produces a waddle-type walk. Similar to the Charlie Chaplin walk when taken to an extreme.	Shoes wear on the back/outer side of the heel.	Pain inside the knee, bunions, arthritis in the knee, and lowback pain.
Toe-In		
Pigeon-toed gait. Kneecaps point inward during stride. Usually takes short steps.	Front of shoes wear on outside. Possible history of ankle sprains.	Hip and ankle pain; may develop eventual arthritis.

Toe-Walk (Bop Gait)

Bouncy stride with short heel contact.	Heavy callouses on balls of feet.	Leg and shin pain; pain in calves of legs; potential for lower back problems.

Stooped Gait

Stooped walk with shuffling of feet.	Poor posture. Round shouldered with head tilted downward when walking.	Chronic low back problems; easily fatigues during walking; instability common in senior citizens with these problems.

Sway Gait

A sauntering stride featuring pronounced sway with movement in either upper body and/or hips. (Think of John Wayne's swagger)	Excessive head movement from side to side when walking.	Associated with much postural difficulty. TMJ, low back pain, and pain with standing.

Source: Howard J. Dananberg, D.P.M., *New Body*, May 1990. Reprinted with permission.

In most of the problematic gaits, myofascial trigger points can also result.

Yes, that pain in your jaw can start at your feet. In learning about your TMJ disorder, you have worked your way from the top of your head all the way down to your feet. And when you think about it, you have also worked from the inside out. I hope that this book has convinced you that you must consider all aspects of your being in designing a plan for a lifetime of good health. It will be your plan, you know, because nobody can do it for you. I hope you will follow in the footsteps of my patients who have taken this very information and made it a part of their lives.

Appendices

A

Recommended Reading

American Heart Association. 1995. *The Healthy Heart Walking Book.* New York: MacMillan Health.
This is an all-around good book for maintaining a healthy heart.

Butler, S. J. 1996. *Conquering Carpal Tunnel Syndrome and Other Repetitive Strain Injuries.* Oakland, Calif.: New Harbinger Publications.
Having spent her career specializing in the correction of soft-tissue injuries, Sharon J. Butler created the program in this book after developing carpal tunnel syndrome herself in 1991. Not only did she completely eliminate her own symptoms of repetitive strain injury, but she also has helped hundreds of others achieve the same relief, non-invasively, permanently, and inexpensively.

Carper, J. 1996. *Stop Aging Now!* New York: HarperCollins.
If you are over eighteen years of age, you are beginning to age and need this complete and up-to-date book on vitamins, minerals, and all the nutrients we need for good health.

DeGood, D. 1997. *The Headache and Neck Pain Workbook.* Oakland, Calif.: New Harbinger Publications.
This is a comprehensive book on headaches that helps readers sort out and overcome head and neck pain.

Gelb, H. 1980. *Killing Pain Without Prescription: A New And Simple Way to Free Yourself From Headache, Backache, and Other Sources of Chronic Pain.* New York: Harper and Row.

This is a book about muscular pain—the kind of pain that is responsible for 90 percent of our aches, according to Gelb. He discusses headaches, backaches, neck aches, and pain of a muscular nature that occurs throughout the body. He tells the reader how to identify the source of the pain and what to do about it, without taking medications that mask the pain.

McKay, M., and P. Fanning. 1997. *The Daily Relaxer.* Oakland, Calif.: New Harbinger Publications.

The focus in this book is on the most effective and popular techniques for learning how to relax. Each relaxer presents a simple, tension-relieving exercise that can be learned in five minutes and practiced with positive results right away.

McKenzie, R. 1997. *Treat Your Own Neck.* New Zealand: Spinal Publications.

———. 1997. *Treat Your Own Back.* New Zealand: Spinal Publications.

Robin McKenzie, world-renowned physiotherapist from Wellington, New Zealand, developed self-treatment programs for people with neck and back problems. He wrote these two easy-to-read books to guide people in their efforts to attain and maintain healthy and pain-free necks and backs. I recommend these books to most of my TMJ patients because the total body is so deeply involved in the diagnosis and treatment of TMJ disorder. To order, call (800) 367-7393 (U.S. and Canada). For more information call (612) 553-0452 or write OPTP, P.O. Box 47009, Minneapolis, MN 55447-0009.

Napier, K. M. 1995. *How Nutrition Works.* Emeryville, Calif.: Ziff-Davis.

This is a colorful, comprehensive, and complete guide to proper nutrition. It is excellent for children as well as adults.

Olson, K. 1989. *The Art of Staying Well in an Uptight World.* Nashville, Tenn.: Oliver Nelson Books.

Ken Olson focuses on helping people develop a healthy lifestyle. He tells why we need to understand the relationship between emotional, mental, spiritual, and physical health and healing. I recommend this book to my patients because of his thorough understanding of TMJ disorder, referred pain, trigger points, and the role stress plays in the healing process.

Prudden, B. 1982. *Pain Erasure: The Bonnie Prudden Way: Discover the Wonders of "Trigger Point" Therapy.* New York: Ballantine Books.

This book provides pain relief through learning about trigger points—what they are, how to deactivate them, and how to prevent their return. This therapy requires no special training or equipment and enjoys a high rate of success.

————. 1984. *Myotherapy: Bonnie Prudden's Complete Guide to Pain-Free Living.* New York: Ballantine Books.

This book is an extension of her previous book and goes on to provide instructions on the "Quick Fix" for immediate pain relief. Prudden also prescribes a complete program called the "Permanent Fix" for a lifetime program of pain-free living.

Schatz, M. P. 1992. *Back Care Basics: A Doctor's Gentle Yoga Program for Back and Neck Pain Relief.* Berkeley, Calif.: Rodmell Press.

This is a book for those interested in gentle yoga. Many of the back exercises recommended by physical therapists and others are derived from yoga techniques. This book offers daily exercise routines to correct the source of back and neck pain.

Starlanyl, D., and M. E. Copeland. 1996. *Fibromyalgia & Chronic Myofascial Pain Syndrome: A Survival Manual.* Oakland, Calif.: New Harbinger Publications.

This is the most comprehensive analysis of fibromyalgia and chronic myofascial pain syndrome available today. It is designed not only to help the patients with these perplexing problems, but also to inform the health professionals working on their behalf.

B

Glossary

Acute. An *acute* disease has a rapid onset, a short duration, and pronounced symptoms. An *acute* pain is sharp and severe.

Ataxia. Loss of the ability to coordinate muscular movement. Unintentional veering while walking, with loss of motor coordination, which can happen unexpectedly.

Atrophy. A wasting or decrease in size of a bodily organ, tissue, or part owing to disease, injury, or lack of use.

Biofeedback. Using machines that measure the skin's electrical response and temperature as well as muscle tension and heartbeat, therapists teach people how to control body functions such as blood pressure, heart rate, and jaw tension.

Bruxism. The habit of grinding your teeth while clenching.

Chronic. Long standing, as opposed to acute.

Chiropractic. A therapy based on the premise that disease is caused by abnormal function of the nervous system. Involves manipulation and treatment of the structures of the body, especially the spinal cord.

Condyle. A rounded prominence at the end of a bone, most often for articulation with another bone. In this book the *condyle* refers to the top of the lower jaw bone.

Disc. This refers to the soft disc that lies between the condyle and temporal bone, in front of the ear bones.

Degenerative joint disease. Chronic degeneration of the cartilage of the joint.

Dysfunction. Abnormal or impaired functioning, especially of a bodily system or organ.

Endorphins. The body's own natural painkillers. They are a brain chemical with a composition remarkably similar to morphine.

Etiological. Assignment of a cause, origin, or reason for something; for example, the cause or origin of a disease or disorder as determined by a medical diagnosis.

Fascia. A sheet of connective tissue that extends without interruption from the top of the head to the tip of toes. It surrounds and invades every other tissue and organ of the body.

Fibromyalgia Syndrome (FMS). A chronic, non-degenerative, non-progressive truly systematic pain condition.

Forward head posture. Posture in which, when viewed from the side of the body, the ear is in front of the center of the shoulder joint.

Inflammation. A localized protective reaction of tissue to irritation, injury, or infection, characterized by pain, redness, localized fever, swelling, and sometimes loss of function.

Internal derangement. The diagnosis whereby the temporomandibular joint is not functioning properly because the codylar disc has been displaced.

Ligaments. Dense bands of connective tissue (collagen) that connect one bone to another.

Lordosis. The natural curve of the spine. The cervical (neck) and lumbar (lower back) areas curve inward, and the thoracic area (middle of back) is slightly rounded out. All three areas need to be properly aligned and balanced.

Magnetic Resonance Imaging (MRI). The use of a nuclear magnetic resonance spectrometer to produce electronic images of specific atoms and molecular structures in solids, especially human cells, tissues, and organs.

Malocclusion. Faulty contact between the upper and lower teeth when the jaw is closed.

Manage (versus "to treat"). To manage is to direct the affairs or interests of patient. To treat requires administration or application of remedies to a patient or for a disease or an injury.

Mandible. The lower jaw.

Massage. The rubbing or kneading of parts of the body to aid circulation or relax the muscles. Works by increasing blood circulation to the soft tissues, helping them heal with oxygen and nutrients.

Myalgia. Muscular pain or tenderness, especially when diffuse and nonspecific.

Maxilla. Either of a pair of bones of the human skull fusing in the midline and forming the upper jaw.

Musculoskeletal. Pertaining to or comprising the skeleton and muscles; as musculoskeletal system.

Myotherapy. A therapy whereby you (1) locate your trigger points, (2) apply seven seconds of pressure where it hurts, and (3) stretch the affected muscles with simple exercises.

Myofascial Release (MFR). An extremely mild and gentle form of stretching used by some physical therapists. It involves positions and stretches that mimic the body's attempt to self-correct its dysfunction. It is a whole-body approach to treatment. The trained therapist has a thorough understanding of the fascial system.

Myofascial trigger points. A hyperirritable spot usually within a taut band of skeletal muscle or the muscles fascia that is painful on compression and can give rise to characteristic referred pain, tenderness, and autonomic phenomena.

Neuromuscular. Having to do with the muscles that move the body and the nerves that coordinate their activity.

Orthotic. A specialized mechanical device to support or supplement weakened or abnormal joints or limbs.

Osteoarthritis. A form of arthritis, occurring mainly in older persons, that is characterized by chronic degeneration of the cartilage of the joints. Also called *degenerative joint disease.*

Osteopathy. A system of medicine based on the theory that disturbance in the musculoskeletal system affects other bodily parts, causing many disorders that can be corrected by various manipulative techniques in conjunction with conventional medical, surgical, pharmacological, and other therapeutic procedures.

Palpable band. A tight muscle in spasm that can be felt.

Passive stretching. A gentle, sustained stretching of the muscle fibers, ligaments, and tendons, as opposed to ballistic, or rapid stretching.

Perpetuating factor. Faulty habit that keeps the TMJ disorder going, such as gum chewing, clenching, poor posture, faulty diet, lack of proper exercise.

Physical therapy. The treatment of physical dysfunction or injury by the use of therapeutic exercise and the application of modalities, intended to restore or facilitate normal function or development. Also called *physiotherapy*. Treatment is performed by a professionally trained physical therapist (often referred to as a P.T.).

Precipitating factor. An event, such as a blow to the head, an auto accident, surgery, or even a wide yawn, that sets off your TMJ disorder.

Predisposing factor. An event or condition that occurs at birth or early in life and sets the stage for future TMJ disorder problems, such as jaw malformation, thumb sucking, early accident, severe illness or bodily abnormaility such as a short leg.

Referred pain. Pain that is felt in one area of the body, but is caused by a trigger point in a muscle in another part of the body.

Relaxation breath. A simple yoga breathing technique in which you pause for one to three seconds at the end of each normal exhalation, then inhale normally.

Rheumatic disorders. Rheumatic disorder or disease is any of several pathological conditions of the muscles, tendons, joints, bones, or nerves, characterized by discomfort and disability.

Scoliosis. An abnormal side-to-side (lateral) curvature of the spine.

Splint. A removeable appliance dentists have used for years to manage TMJ disorder. The appliance has a flat acrylic (hard plastic) pad that covers the lower or upper teeth relieving pressure in the jaw joint.

Syndrome. A specific set of signs and symptoms that occur together.

Temporal. Of, relating to, or near the temples of the skull.

Tender point. Specific spots on the body that cause pain when pressure is applied to the area.

Tendons. A band of tough, inelastic fibrous tissue that connects a muscle with its bony attachment.

Trigger point. See Myofascial trigger point.

Trigger-point therapy. The therapist applies concentrated finger pressure to trigger points to break the cycle of spasm and pain.

Vertigo. A sensation of dizziness; a confused, disorientated state of mind.

Yoga. The ancient philosophical and therapeutic system developed in India to encourage harmonious living and mental and physical health. It involves postures, exercises, breathing techniques, and meditation.

References

Baltzell, J. 1990. *Stress Reduction at the Healing Center*. Chanhassen, Minn.: J. Baltzell. A pamphlet.

———. 1993. *Yoga at the Healing Center*. Chanhassen, Minn.: J. Baltzell. A pamphlet.

Barnes, J. F. 1990. *Myofascial Release: The Search for Excellence—A Comprehensive Evaluatory and Treatment Approach*. Paoli, Penn.: MFR Publications.

———. 1995. Myofascial Release: The "missing link" in your treatment. *Physical Therapy Today* January 16.

Bennett, R. M. 1997. Fibromyalgia Review. *Journal of Musculoskeletal Pain* 5(4):71–86.

Brady, C., D. Taylor, and M. O'Brien. 1993. Whiplash and temporomandibular joint dysfunction. *Journal of the Irish Dental Ass'n* 39(3).

Burgess, J. 1991. Symptom characteristics in TMD patients reporting blunt trauma and/or whiplash injury. *Journal of Craniomandibular Disorders: Facial & Oral Pain* 5(4):251–256.

Buskiila, D., L. Neumann, G. Vaisberg, D. Alkalay, and F. Wolfe. 1997. Increased rates of fibromyalgia following cervical spine injury: A controlled study of 161 cases of traumatic injury. *Arthritis and Rheumatism* 39:446–452.

Butler, J. 1996. *Conquering Carpal Tunnel Syndrome and Other Repetitive Strain Injuries.* Oakland, Calif.: New Harbinger Publications.

Cirbus, M. T., M. S. Smilack, J. Beltran, and D. C. Simons. 1997. Magnetic resonance imaging in confirming internal derangement of the temporomandibular joint. *Journal of Prosthetic Dentistry* 57(4): 35–45.

Croft, A. C. 1992. The cervical acceleration/deceleration syndrome. In *Whiplash and Temporomandibular Disorders: An Interdisciplinary Approach to Case Management,* edited by D. P. Steigerwald and A. C. Croft. Encinita, Calif.: Encinita Kaiser.

Dananberg, H. J. 1990. It's all in the stride. *New Body.*

———. 1993. Gait style as an etiology to chronic postural pain. Part I: Functional hallus limitus. *Journal of the American Podiatric Medical Association* 83(8):433–441.

———. 1993. Gait style as an etiology to chronic postural pain. Part II: Postural compensatory process. *Journal of the American Podiatric Medical Association* 83(11):615–624.

Davis, A. 1954. *Let's Eat Right to Keep Fit.* New York: Harcourt and Bruce Co.

Epstein, J. B. 1992. Temporomandibular disorders, facial pain and headache following motor vehicle accidents. *Journal Canadian Dental Association* 58(6).

Farrar, W. B., and W. L. McCarty, Jr. 1982. *A Clinical Outline of Temporomandibular Joint Diagnoses and Treatment.* Montgomery, Ala.: Montgomery Walker Printing Co.

Farrar, W. B., W. L. McCarty, Jr., and J. Witzig. 1979. *Clicking.* St. Paul, Minn.: European Orthodontic Products.

Fricton, J. R., R. J. Kroening, and K. M. Hathaway. 1988. *TMJ and Craniofascial Pain: Diagnosis and Management*. St. Louis, Mo., and Tokyo: Ishiyaku EuroAmerica, Inc.

Garcia, R. Jr., and J. A. Arrington. 1996. The relationship between cervical whiplash and TMJ injuries: An MRI study. *CRANIO: The Journal of Craniomandibular Practice* 14(3):233–239.

Gelb, H. 1977. *Clinical Management of Head, Neck, and TMJ Pain and Dysfunction: A Multidisciplinary Approach to Diagnosis and Treatment*. Philadelphia: W.B. Saunders Co.

———. 1980. *Killing Pain Without Prescription*. New York: Harper and Row.

Greene, C. S. 1992. Managing TMD patients: Initial therapy is the key. *Journal of the American Dental Association (JADA)* 123:43–45.

Hathaway, K. 1984. Non-stress-related clenching, bruxism, and other habits. University of Minnesota, Minn. A handout.

———. 1997. Evaluation and management of maladaptive behaviors and psychological issues in temporomandibular disorder patients. *Dental Clinics of North America* 41(2):341–354.

Kinnie, B. H. 1982. Whiplash trauma: Treatment responsibility. *The Whiplash Mechanism in Traumatic Injury*. Columbia, S.C. A pamphlet.

Kronn, E. 1993. The incidence of TMJ dysfunction in patients who have suffered a cervical whiplash injury following a traffic accident. *Journal of Orofacial Pain* 7:209–213.

Lader, E. 1983. *TMJ: A Comprehensive Systems Manual*. Dix Hills, N.Y.: Valdare Publishing.

Levine, J. D, M. S. Gordon, and H. L. Fields. 1978. The mechanism of placebo analgesia. *The Lancet* 2:654–657.

McKenzie, R. 1997. *Treat Your Own Back*. Waikanae, New Zealand: Spinal Publications New Zealand Ltd.

———. 1997. *Treat Your Own Neck*. Waikanae, New Zealand: Spinal Publications New Zealand Ltd.

National Institute of Dental Research. TMD: Temporomandibluar Disorders (publication no. 94-3487). Washington, D. C.: NIH Publication.

Prudden, B. 1977. *Pain Erasure: The Bonnie Prudden Way*. New York: Ballantine Books.

———. 1984. *Myotherapy: Bonnie Prudden's Complete Guide to Pain-Free Living*. New York: Ballantine Books.

Rocabado, M. 1983. *Basic Exercises for Initial Postural Correction of the Jaw, Head, and Neck*. A handout.

———. 1983. Arthokinetics of the TMJ. *Dent. Clinics of N. Am.* 27:573–591.

Rogal, O. J. 1988. *Mandibular Whiplash*. Philadelphia: The TMJ Dental Trauma Center for Head, Facial & Neck Pain.

Selye, H. 1956. *The Stress of Life*. New York: McGraw Hill.

Shore, N. A. 1959. *Occlusal Equilibration and TMJ Dysfunction*. Philadelphia: J. B. Lippincott Co.

Simons, D. G. 1987. *Myofascial Pain Syndrome Due to Trigger Points*. IRMA (International Rehabilitation Medicine Association). Monograph Series 1. Cleveland, Ohio: Rademaker Printing.

———. 1993. Referred phenomenon of myofascial trigger points. In *New Trends in Referred Pain and Hyperalgesia*. New York: Elsevier Science Publishers, B.V.

———. 1996. Clinical and etiological update of myofascial pain from trigger points. *Journal of Musculoskeletal Pain* 4:93–121.

———. 1997. Myofascial trigger points: The critical experiment. *Journal of Musculoskeletal Pain* 5(4):113–118.

Slavkin, H. 1997. Chronic disabling diseases and disorders: The challenge of fibromyalgia. *The Journal of the American Dental Association* 128:1583–1589.

Smith, S. 1981. *Atlas of Temporomandibular Orthopedics*. Philadelphia: Philadelphia College of Osteopathic Medicine Press.

Starlanyl, D., and M. E. Copeland. 1996. *Fibromyalgia & Chronic Myofascial Pain: A Survival Manual*. Oakland, Calif.: New Harbinger Publications.

Starlanyl, D. 1997. *Chronic Myofascial Pain Syndrome: A Guide to the Trigger Points* (a videotape). Oakland, Calif.: New Harbinger Publications.

Travell, J. 1960: Temporomandibular joint referred pain from the muscles of the head and neck. *Journal of Prosthetic Dentistry* 10(4):745–763.

Travell, J. G., and D. G. Simons. 1983. *Myofascial Pain and Dysfunction: The Trigger Point Manual*, Vol. 1. Baltimore, Md.: Williams and Wilkens.

———. 1993. *The Trigger Point Manual*, Vol. 2. Baltimore, Md.: Williams and Wilkens.

Uppgaard, R. O. 1978. Diagnosis and treatment of head and face pain. *Northwest Dentistry* Sept-Oct:295–298.

———. 1992. Conservative and successful treatment of TMJ dysfunction in private rural practice. *CRANIO: The Journal of Craniomandibular Practice* 10(3):235–240.

Witzig, J. 1994. *How to Treat TMJ Patients Successfully Including the Four Essentials For Successful TMJ Treatment of Injured Joints*. Minneapolis, Minn.: TMJ Institute of America.

Wright, E. F., K. F. DeRosier, M. K. Clark, and S. L. Bifano. 1997. Identifying undiagnosed rheumatic disorders among patients with TMD. *Journal of the American Dental Association* 128:738–744.

Index

A

acute, defined, 163

American Medical Association (AMA), 3, 135

anterior bite planes, 146

arm circles, 111

arm stretch, 111

Art of Staying Well in an Uptight World, The (Olson), 160

assessment: of harmful habits, 28–29, 75–77; of pain patterns, 31–33; of stressors, 87–89. *See also* self-assessment of TMJ disorder

asthma, 85

ataxia, 163

Atlas of Temporomandibular Orthopedics, The (Smith), 62

atrophy, 163

axial extension of the neck exercise, 44

B

Back Care Basics: A Doctor's Gentle Yoga Program for Back and Neck Pain Relief (Schatz), 161

back stretch exercises, 73–74, 112

back support, 71

Baltzell, James, 107

Barnes, John, 16, 57, 151

biofeedback, 154, 163

biotin, 101

blood vessels, related to temporomandibular joints, 14–15

body: assessing pain patterns throughout, 32–33; fascia in, 16–17; listening to, 89–90; myofascia in, 17–18; symptoms of TMJ disorder in, 24

bop gait, 156

bruxism, 163

C

calcium, 101

cardiovascular disease, 84

cat stretch, 115

causes and contributing factors: of fibromyalgia syndrome, 135–136; of TMJ disorder, 19–21

cervical collars, 130

cervical lordosis, 63

cervical traction, 130

cervical whiplash, 2, 121; common symptoms of, 125–126

changing harmful habits, 75–80

cheek muscle, 51–52

chiropractic, 152–153, 163

chronic, defined, 163

clenching: exercise for avoiding, 37; jaw problems and, 35–36

clicking noises, 23

coexisting conditions: fibromyalgia syndrome, 139–140; self-assessment questionnaire for, 26–27

communicating with physicians, 5

Comprehensive Systems Manual, A (Lader), 128

condyles, 13, 163

Conquering Carpal Tunnel Syndrome and Other Repetitive Strain Injuries (Butler), 159

contributing factors. *See* causes and contributing factors

control TMJ rotation exercise, 41

coping strategies for stress, 85–93; assessing your stressors, 87–89; getting enough sleep, 91–93; learning deep breathing techniques, 90; listening to your body, 89–90; organizing your time, 89; setting priorities, 86–87

copper, 101

Croft, Arthur C., 127

cyanocobalamin, 100

D

Daily Relaxer, The (McKay and Fanning), 89, 160

Dananberg, Howard J., 154–155

Davis, Adele, 95

deep breathing, 90

degenerative joint disease, 15, 164

delayed onset of TMJ disorder, 127–129

dental causes of TMJ disorder, 19

diagnosis: of fibromyalgia syndrome, 136–138; of TMJ disorder, 24–33

dietary habits. *See* nutritional habits

disc, 13, 163

doorway stretch, 116

driving posture, 70–71

duck toe gait, 155

dysfunction, defined, 164

E

eating habits. *See* nutritional habits

emotional causes of TMJ disorder, 20

endorphins, 164

etiological, defined, 164

exercise habits, 95–96, 106–117; general guidelines for, 106; recommended stretching exercises, 108–117; rules for stretching and, 108; yoga exercise and, 107. *See also* nutritional habits

exercises to improve jaw functioning, 35–44; avoiding clenching, 37; axial extension of the neck, 44; controlling TMJ rotation, 41; head and neck stretch, 41–42; improving

shoulder posture, 43; increasing the jaw opening, 39; rhythmic stabilization, 40; stabilization head flexion, 43–44; stretching the jaw, 38

F

facial feature imbalance, 30–31

Fanning, Patrick, 89

fascia, 16–17, 164

feature imbalance, 30–31

Fibromyalgia & Chronic Myofascial Pain Syndrome (Starlanyl and Copeland), 137, 161

fibromyalgia syndrome (FMS), 3, 133–140; causes of, 135–136; compared to TMJ disorder, 138–139; defined, 164; diagnosis of, 136–138; explanation of, 135; symptoms of, 136; treatment for, 138

fight-or-flight response, 84

flexion/extension exercise, 114

FMS. *See* fibromyalgia syndrome

folic acid, 100

foot problems, 154–156

forward head posture, 164

F-S Index of the Craniomandibular Pain Syndrome, 21, 22

functional hallux limitus (FHL), 155

Funt, Lawrence, 4, 20

G

gait, style of, 155–156

gastrointestinal problems, 85

Gelb, Harold, 4, 144

glossary of terms, 163–167

grating noises, 23

Greene, Charles S., 5, 147

Guide to Good Eating (USDA), 96–98

H

hamstring stretch, 112, 114

harmful habits, 59–80; breaking, 75–80; lack of exercise, 95–96; muscle abuse, 74; nighttime, 62; nutritional, 74, 96–105; oral, 60–62; postural, 62–74; self-assessment of, 28–29, 75–77; TMJ disorder caused by, 20, 28–29

hatha yoga, 153

Hathaway, Kate, 60, 79

head: assessing pain patterns in, 31–32; pain referral patterns from, 48–55; stretching exercises, 41–42, 43–44; symptoms of TMJ disorder in, 24

head and neck circles, 112

Headache and Neck Pain Workbook, The (DeGood), 159

head-on collisions, 124

health: exercise habits and, 95–96, 106–117; nutritional habits and, 74, 95–105; prolonged stress and, 84–85

health history checklist, 27–29

Healthy Heart Walking Book, The (AHA), 159

heel-toe gait, 155

home remedies, 57

How Nutrition Works (Napier), 160

Hultgren, Dale, 152

I

immune system, 84

increasing the jaw opening exercise, 39

inflammation, 164

injuries: as cause of TMJ disorder, 2, 19; intensity of impact and, 127. *See also* whiplash injuries

insomnia, 91–92

internal derangement, 15, 18, 143, 164

iron, 102

J

jaw: exercises to improve functioning of, 35–44; internal derangement of, 15, 18; symptoms of TMJ disorder in, 21, 23; temporomandibular joints and, 13–15; visual self-examination of, 30–31

Jump Sign, 47

K

Killing Pain Without Prescription (Gelb), 160

Kinnie, Bruce H., 123

kneeling pectoral stretch, 115

knee-to-chest exercise, 114

L

Lader, Errol, 128

lateral pterygoid, 53–54

legs-up-the-wall exercise, 116

levator scapulae, 55

lifting posture, 65

ligaments, 164

lordosis, 63, 164

lower repositioning splints, 146

lumbar lordosis, 63

M

macrotraumas, 61

magnesium, 102

magnetic resonance imaging (MRI), 130, 164

malocclusion, 164

mandible, 13, 165

mandibular orthopedic repositioning appliance (MORA), 142, 144–145. *See also* splints

mandibular whiplash, 2, 121; common symptoms of, 125–126

massage, 165

masseter, 51–52

maxilla, 165

McKay, Matthew, 89

McKenzie, Robin, 63

mechanical stresses, 28

medial pterygoid, 53

microtraumas, 61

minerals, 99; chart of required, 101–103; documenting your deficiencies, 103–104; taking as supplements, 104–105

modified sit-up, 113

MORA. *See* mandibular orthopedic repositioning appliance

Morin, Charles M., 91

motor vehicle accidents (MVAs), 2, 123–125, 127

mountain pose, 109–110

MRI (magnetic resonance imaging), 130, 164

muscles: abuse of, 29, 74, 77; myofascia and, 17–18; referred pain and, 46–57; related to TMJ disorder, 13–14

musculoskeletal, defined, 165

myalgia, 165

myofascia, 17–18

myofascial pain, 15, 16–18, 143

Myofascial Pain and Dysfunction: The Trigger Point Manual (Travell and Simons), 46

Myofascial Release (MFR), 16, 57, 122, 151–152, 165

myofascial trigger points. *See* trigger points

Myotherapy, 56, 152, 165

Myotherapy: Bonnie Prudden's Complete Guide to Pain-Free Living, 161

myths about whiplash injuries, 126–131

N

napping, 92–93

National Institute of Dental Research (NIDR), 15, 130

neck: assessing pain patterns in, 31–32; axial extension of, 44; pain referral patterns from, 48–55; stretching exercises, 41–42, 43–44

nerves, related to temporomandibular joints, 14–15

neuromuscular, defined, 165

niacin, 99

nighttime oral habits, 62

nutritional habits, 74, 95–106; food groups guide and, 96–98;

improving, 104–105; self-assessment of, 29, 77, 96–104; TMJ disorder caused by, 20; vitamin/mineral consumption and, 99–104. *See also* exercise habits

O

occlusal habits. *See* oral habits

Olson, Ken, 87

oral habits, 60–62; breaking harmful habits, 79; nighttime, 62; self- assessment of, 28, 75–76; TMJ disorder caused by, 20

orthotics, 142, 165. *See also* splints

osteoarthritis, 165

osteopathy, 165

P

pain: around the head and neck, 31–32; referred from trigger points, 46–57; therapies for relieving, 56–57; throughout the body, 32–33

Pain Erasure: The Bonnie Prudden Way, 56, 161

Palmer, D. D., 152

palpable band, 166

pantothenic acid, 101

passive stretching, 166

pectoral stretch, 113

pelvic tilt, 113

perpetuating factors, 27, 28–29, 166

phone holding position, 68

phosphorus, 102

physical therapy, 56, 150–151, 166

physiological rest position, 144

pigeon-toed gait, 155

podiatry treatment, 154–156

postural habits, 62–74; back stretch exercise and, 73–74; exercises for improving, 43, 44; self-assessment of, 28–29, 76–77; sitting posture, 66–72; sleeping posture, 72–73; standing posture, 63–66; TMJ disorder caused by, 20

potassium, 102

precipitating factors, 27, 28, 166

predisposing factors, 27–28, 166

priority setting, 86–87

Prudden, Bonnie, 56

psychological stresses, 29

pyridoxine, 100

Q

questionnaires. *See* self-assessment of TMJ disorder

R

reading in bed, 70

rear-end collisions, 123–124

recommended reading on TMJ disorder, 159–161

referred pain, 45–57; defined, 166; steps for easing, 48–49; therapies for relieving, 56–57; trigger points and, 46–55

relaxation breathing, 90, 166

rheumatic disorders, 133–134, 166

rhythmic stabilization exercise, 40

riboflavin, 99

Rocabado, Mariano, 35, 150

rounded back posture, 67

S

scoliosis, 166

selenium, 102

self-assessment of TMJ disorder, 24–33; coexisting conditions questionnaire, 26–27; harmful habits and, 28–29, 75–77; health history checklist, 27–29; pain pattern assessment, 31–33; stressors and, 87–88; symptoms checklist, 25–26; visual exam, 30–31

setting priorities, 86–87

shoulder rolls, 110

shoulder shrug, 110

shoulders: pain referral patterns from, 48–55; postural improvement exercise for, 43

Simons, David, 4, 46, 47, 125

sitting posture, 66–72; after vigorous activity, 72; on the couch, 69; driving, 70–71; holding the phone, 68; reading in bed, 70; rounded back, 67–68; sleeping in a chair, 68–69; without back support, 71

sleep, 91–93; insomnia and, 91–92; napping and, 92–93; requirements for, 91

sleep deprivation, 91

sleeping posture, 72–73; in a chair, 68–69

Smith, Steven, 62

social causes of TMJ disorder, 20

spine roll, 115

splenius cervicus, 49

splints, 141–147; defined, 142, 166; how they work, 144–147; need for using, 143; reasons for using, 142–143; whiplash injuries and, 130–131

spot tenderness, 47

Spray and Stretch technique, 56

stabilization head flexion exercise, 43–44

Stack, Brendan, 20

standing posture, 63–66; lifting and, 65; walking and, 64; working in stooped positions, 65–66

Stein, William E., 146

sternocleidomastoid (SCM), 50

stooped gait, 156

stooped working positions, 65–66

Stop Aging Now! (Carper), 159

stress, 81–93; coping strategies for, 85–93; defined, 82; facial muscles related to, 14; health problems and, 84–85; major causes of, 83; physiological response to, 84; TMJ disorder and, 20, 81

stressors, 82; assessing, 87–89; life events as, 83

stress-response mechanism, 84

stretching: the jaw muscles, 38; recommended program of, 109–117; rules about, 108; yoga exercise and, 107

sway gait, 156

symptoms: of fibromyalgia syndrome, 136, 139; of TMJ disorder, 21–24, 139; of whiplash injuries, 125–126

syndrome, defined, 166

T

temporal, defined, 166

temporal bone, 13

temporalis, 54–55

temporomandibular joint disorder. *See* TMJ disorder

temporomandibular joints, 13; blood vessels related to, 14–15; illustrated, 14; muscles related to, 13–14; nerves related to, 14–15 tender points, 136–138, 166. *See also* trigger points

tendons, 167

therapies. *See* treatment options

thiamine, 99

time management, 89

TMJ disorder: blood vessels related to, 14–15; causes of, 19–21; fibromyalgia syndrome and, 3, 133–140; glossary of terms associated with, 163–167; muscles related to, 13–14; names for, 2; nerves related to, 14–15; recommended reading on, 159–161; self-assessment of, 24–33; splints used for, 141–147; statistics on, 2; symptoms of, 21–24; treatment options for, 149–156; types of, 15–18; whiplash and, 2, 121–131

toe-walk (bop gait), 156

Total Wellness Program: development and success of, 3–4; eliminating harmful habits, 59–80; evaluating/improving exercise habits, 95–96, 106–117; evaluating/improving nutritional habits, 95–105; identifying stressors, 81–93; jaw-related exercises, 35–44; personal understanding phase, 11–33; treating referred trigger point pain, 45–57

trapezius, 51

Travell, Janet, 4, 46, 125

Treat Your Own Back (McKenzie), 63, 160

Treat Your Own Neck (McKenzie), 63, 160

treatment options, 149–156; biofeedback, 154; chiropractic, 152–153; Myofascial Release, 16, 57, 122, 151–152; Myotherapy, 56, 152; physical therapy, 56, 150–151; podiatry treatment, 154–156; yoga exercise, 107, 153–154

trigger points (TrPs), 45–57; defined, 165; lateral pterygoid, 53–54; levator scapulae, 55; locating, 48; masseter, 51–52; medial pterygoid, 53; referred pain from, 46–55; splenius cervicus, 49; sternocleidomastoid, 50; temporalis, 54–55; therapies for relieving, 56–57; trapezius, 51. *See also* tender points

trigger-point therapy, 56, 167

U

University of Minnesota TMJ and Craniofacial Pain Clinic, 4

upper back stretch, 111

upper (maxillary) flat bite plane splints, 146

V

vertigo, 167

visual examination, 30–31

vitamins: chart of required, 99–101; documenting your deficiencies, 103–104; taking as supplements, 104–105

W

walking posture, 64

whiplash injuries, 2, 121–131; common myths about, 126–131; explanation of, 123–125; symptoms of, 125–126

working postures: rounded back, 67–68; stooped positions, 65–66

Wright, Edward, 26

X

X rays, 129–130

Y

yoga, 107, 153–154, 167

Z

zinc, 103

More New Harbinger
Self-Help Titles

THE CHRONIC PAIN CONTROL WORKBOOK

A team of specialists in all areas of pain management detail the treatment strategies for managing and recovering from chronic pain.

Item PN2 $18.95

FIBROMYALGIA & CHRONIC MYOFASCIAL PAIN SYNDROME

This survival manual is the first comprehensive patient guide for managing these conditions. Readers learn how to identify trigger points, cope with chronic pain and sleep problems, and deal with the numbing effects of "fibrofog."

Item FMS $19.95

THE HEADACHE AND NECK PAIN WORKBOOK

Combines the latest research with proven alternative therapies to help sufferers of head and neck pain understand and master their condition.

Item NECK $14.95

CONQUERING CARPAL TUNNEL SYNDROME

Guided by symptom charts, you select the best exercises for restoring the range of motion to overworked hands and arms.

Item CARP $17.95

PREPARING FOR SURGERY

Details tested techniques to prepare the mind and body for surgery—techniques that have been found to help decrease the need for postoperative pain medicine, reduce complications, and promote a quicker return to health.

Item PREP, $17.95

THE RELAXATION & STRESS REDUCTION WORKBOOK

Step-by-step instructions cover all of the most effective and popular techniques for learning how to relax.

Item RS4, $17.95

Call **toll-free 1-800-748-6273** to order. Have your Visa or Mastercard number ready. Or send a check for the titles you want to New Harbinger Publications, 5674 Shattuck Avenue, Oakland, CA 94609. Include $3.80 for the first book and 75¢ for each additional book to cover shipping and handling. (California residents please include appropriate sales tax.) Allow four to six weeks for delivery.

Prices subject to change without notice.

Some Other New Harbinger Self-Help Titles

Claiming Your Creative Self: True Stories from the Everyday Lives of Women, $15.95
Six Keys to Creating the Life You Desire, $19.95
Taking Control of TMJ, $13.95
What You Need to Know About Alzheimer's, $15.95
Winning Against Relapse: A Workbook of Action Plans for Recurring Health and Emotional Problems, $14.95
Facing 30: Women Talk About Constructing a Real Life and Other Scary Rites of Passage, $12.95
The Worry Control Workbook, $15.95
Wanting What You Have: A Self-Discovery Workbook, $18.95
When Perfect Isn't Good Enough: Strategies for Coping with Perfectionism, $13.95
The Endometriosis Survival Guide, $13.95
Earning Your Own Respect: A Handbook of Personal Responsibility, $12.95
High on Stress: A Woman's Guide to Optimizing the Stress in Her Life, $13.95
Infidelity: A Survival Guide, $13.95
Stop Walking on Eggshells, $14.95
Consumer's Guide to Psychiatric Drugs, $16.95
The Fibromyalgia Advocate: Getting the Support You Need to Cope with Fibromyalgia and Myofascial Pain, $18.95
Healing Fear: New Approaches to Overcoming Anxiety, $16.95
Working Anger: Preventing and Resolving Conflict on the Job, $12.95
Sex Smart: How Your Childhood Shaped Your Sexual Life and What to Do About It, $14.95
You Can Free Yourself From Alcohol & Drugs, $13.95
Amongst Ourselves: A Self-Help Guide to Living with Dissociative Identity Disorder, $14.95
Healthy Living with Diabetes, $13.95
Dr. Carl Robinson's Basic Baby Care, $10.95
Better Boundaries: Owning and Treasuring Your Life, $13.95
Goodbye Good Girl, $12.95
Being, Belonging, Doing, $10.95
Thoughts & Feelings, Second Edition, $18.95
Depression: How It Happens, How It's Healed, $14.95
Trust After Trauma, $15.95
The Chemotherapy & Radiation Survival Guide, Second Edition, $14.95
Surviving Childhood Cancer, $12.95
The Headache & Neck Pain Workbook, $14.95
Perimenopause, $16.95
The Self-Forgiveness Handbook, $12.95
A Woman's Guide to Overcoming Sexual Fear and Pain, $14.95
Don't Take It Personally, $12.95
Becoming a Wise Parent For Your Grown Child, $12.95
Clear Your Past, Change Your Future, $13.95
Preparing for Surgery, $17.95
The Power of Two, $15.95
It's Not OK Anymore, $13.95
The Daily Relaxer, $12.95
The Body Image Workbook, $17.95
Living with ADD, $17.95
When Anger Hurts Your Kids, $12.95
The Chronic Pain Control Workbook, Second Edition, $17.95
Fibromyalgia & Chronic Myofascial Pain Syndrome, $19.95
Kid Cooperation: How to Stop Yelling, Nagging & Pleading and Get Kids to Cooperate, $13.95
The Stop Smoking Workbook: Your Guide to Healthy Quitting, $17.95
Conquering Carpal Tunnel Syndrome and Other Repetitive Strain Injuries, $17.95
An End to Panic: Breakthrough Techniques for Overcoming Panic Disorder, Second Edition, $18.95
Letting Go of Anger: The 10 Most Common Anger Styles and What to Do About Them, $12.95
Messages: The Communication Skills Workbook, Second Edition, $15.95
Coping With Chronic Fatigue Syndrome: Nine Things You Can Do, $13.95
The Anxiety & Phobia Workbook, Second Edition, $18.95
The Relaxation & Stress Reduction Workbook, Fourth Edition, $17.95
Living Without Depression & Manic Depression: A Workbook for Maintaining Mood Stability, $18.95
Coping With Schizophrenia: A Guide For Families, $15.95
Visualization for Change, Second Edition, $15.95
Angry All the Time: An Emergency Guide to Anger Control, $12.95
Couple Skills: Making Your Relationship Work, $14.95
Self-Esteem, Second Edition, $13.95
I Can't Get Over It, A Handbook for Trauma Survivors, Second Edition, $16.95
Dying of Embarrassment: Help for Social Anxiety and Social Phobia, $13.95
The Depression Workbook: Living With Depression and Manic Depression, $17.95
Men & Grief: A Guide for Men Surviving the Death of a Loved One, $14.95
When Once Is Not Enough: Help for Obsessive Compulsives, $14.95
Beyond Grief: A Guide for Recovering from the Death of a Loved One, $14.95
Hypnosis for Change: A Manual of Proven Techniques, Third Edition, $15.95
When Anger Hurts, $13.95

Call **toll free, 1-800-748-6273,** to order. Have your Visa or Mastercard number ready. Or send a check for the titles you want to New Harbinger Publications, Inc., 5674 Shattuck Ave., Oakland, CA 94609. Include $3.80 for the first book and 75¢ for each additional book, to cover shipping and handling. (California residents please include appropriate sales tax.) Allow two to five weeks for delivery.

Prices subject to change without notice.